西部农村居民对医疗服务的认知：
基于消费者决策过程理论的实证研究

卞鹰　　　　主编

何馨　苗杨　　副主编

U0239029

山东大学出版社

图书在版编目(CIP)数据

西部农村居民对医疗服务的认知:基于消费者决策
过程理论的实证研究:英文/卞鹰主编.—济南:山
东大学出版社,2020.8
ISBN 978-7-5607-6696-6

Ⅰ.①西… Ⅱ.①卞… Ⅲ.①农村－卫生服务－研究
－西北地区－英文②农村－卫生服务－研究－西南地区－
英文 Ⅳ.①R199.2

中国版本图书馆 CIP 数据核字(2020)第 167112 号

策划编辑 唐 棣
责任编辑 张申华
封面设计 王 艳

出版发行 山东大学出版社
社 址 山东省济南市山大南路 20 号
邮政编码 250100
发行热线 (0531)88363008
经 销 新华书店
印 刷 济南巨丰印刷有限公司
规 格 720 毫米×1000 毫米 1/16
15.25 印张 366 千字
版 次 2020 年 8 月第 1 版
印 次 2020 年 8 月第 1 次印刷
定 价 60.00 元

Preface

With a rapid growth of health expenditure in China, using available healthcare resources in a more efficient and equitable way has become an important issue. Although health care delivery system improvement and universal health insurance have been implemented since the health reform, many backward regions still face the limited accessibility of health resources and inequity of health care performance. Analyzing patient health demand and perception of health care service performance in rural regions is essential for evaluating the overall efficiency and performance of medical services.

Previous studies had explored the Chinese outpatient health seeking behavior and satisfaction in developed areas and tertiary hospitals. Considering the lower education level, less individual income and heavier economic burden, it is necessary to conduct a region-specific questionnaire survey for the outpatient's perception in rural western China. The main framework of the field study was constructed based on the consumer decision process theory, based on which outpatient satisfaction and choice of health care providers and relevant factors were investigated, to explore outpatients' perception of health care provider in rural western China.

Eleven provincial level divisions in western China were chosen as sample provinces, all counties in each province were divided into three levels by GDP per capita, and one sample county were randomly stratified from each level of 11 provinces. The local county general hospital, the county maternal and child health center (MCH), the county hospital of traditional chinese medicine (TCM) in each sample county were chosen as sample county hospitals, and 2-3 township health centers in each sample county were systematical selected as sample township hospitals. Fifty outpatients randomly drawn from each county hospital and 30 patients from each township health center were enrolled into the questionnaire survey. Written informed consent was obtained from all interviewees before filling the questionnaire.

Questionnaire was composed based on the literature review. to survey outpatient choice and satisfaction. Outpatient choice of care providers was explored through a single-choice question, with participant characteristics investigated as internal factors, while external factors were analyzed through a multiple-choice question. Multinomial logistic regression and Chi-Square analysis was conducted to study the relevant factors. Questionnaire composed of nine 5-Likert items was applied to survey the primary health care outpatient satisfaction. Exploratory factor analysis (EFA) was conducted to study the factor structure of questionnaire. Stepwise multi-linear regression analysis was performed to study the influencing factors.

A total of 4,233 participants form 164 healthcare institutions completed the questionnaire. According to the results, township health center was the primary option for nearly half of responders, outpatients with better socioeconomic status cared more about "doctors' and nurses' professional skills" and "staff service attitude", and tended to select higher level hospitals, outpatients who chose village clinics cared more about "hospital distance". Outpatient satisfaction in rural western China was lower than developed areas and tertiary hospitals, "service attitude" "facility and professional skills" and "patients' cost" were the main three dimensions of overall satisfaction, with significant differences among patients with difference demographic characteristics and chronic disease conditions. With the growth of personal income and promotion of universal coverage, the dominant factor in outpatient evaluation would transform from the affordability to the accessibility of high-quality care.

Outpatients' perception and demand of health care in rural western China have their own uniqueness. Different hospitals should fulfill different functions. While the patient perceived health care performance in rural western China is certainly needed to be improved, since the high-performance health care service will become the greatest concentration of patient in backward areas. Local health care providers should assess and manage the outpatient service quality based on the actual need of patients, considering patients' demographic characteristics and health status. While policy makers and care payers should evaluate the service performance of different hospitals based on different standards. Meanwhile, efficient hospital management methods, modern technologies and staff trainings are still needed, to ensure efficient health care delivery and balanced allocation of care resources.

Healthiness education is one of the most vital components of public health. According to its theoretical conceptual framework, three parts, namely knowledge/perception, attitude and practice are the key points of that areas, so it's nominated as KAP model. Therefore, this book is the first one of a book series according to the project design. There follows two studies after the present study, namely "medical attitude measurement of rural population in western China" and "health intervention for practice sustainable changing of rural population in western China". It is hoped that they will be completed within five years.

Contents

Part I Outpatients Study

Part II　Inpatients Study

Part I Outpatients Study

List of Abbreviations

AR	Adjusted residual
CI	Confidence interval
CSQ	Client satisfaction questionnaire
EFA	Exploratory factor analysis
EPR	Electronic patient record
GDP	Gross domestic product
HAQ Index	Health access and quality index
HBM	Health belief model
HCAHPS	Hospital consumer assessment of health care providers and systems
IIC	Inter item correlation
KMO	Kaiser-Meyer-Olkin
MCH	Maternal and child health center
MSA	Measure of sample adequacy
NBSC	National Bureau of Statistics of China
NHC	National Health Commission of PRC
NHFPC	National Health and Family Planning Commission of the PRC
NHSS	National health service survey
NRCMS	New rural cooperative medical scheme
PAPM	Precaution adoption process model
PHC	Primary health care
PJHQ	Patient judgement of hospital quality

PRC	People's Republic of China
PSQ	Patient satisfaction questionnaire
PSS	Patient satisfaction scale
QCPP	Quality of care from the patient's perception
RCMS	Rural cooperative medical system
SD	Standard deviation
SPPCS	Satisfaction with physician and primary care scale
TCM	Traditional Chinese medicine
TRA/TPB	Theory of reasoned action/theory of planned behavior
TTM/SOC	Transtheoretical model/stage of change
UEBMI	Urban employee basic medical insurance
URBMI	Urban resident basic medical insurance
WHO	World Health Organization

Chapter 1 Introduction

1.1 Background

1.1.1 The rapid growth of health expenditure in China

Since the reform and opening-up in 1978, China has made great progress in economy and public health during the past 40 years. With the advances in medical technology and growth of life expectancy, a rapid increase of health expenditure was also observed. (Meng et al., 2012; Tian et al., 2013)

In 2015, the global average healthcare expending per capita was $ 1,001, with an annual growth rate of 2% since 2010, while the health expenditure per capita of high-income countries was $ 5,050, with an annual growth of 1.8% since 2010. (World Bank Group, 2017; see details in Figure 1-1).

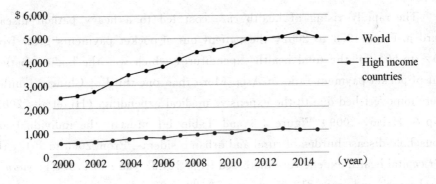

Figure 1-1　Health expenditure of the world and high-income countries (2000-2015)

Although the health expenses in China is still below the global average, which however increased much faster in the past few years. According to the World Bank data (World Bank Group, 2017), the Gross Domestic Product (GDP) per capital in China had reached more than $4,382 in 2010, which means China became an upper middle-income country. As shown in Figure 1-2, in 2010 the health expenditure per capita in China was $199, almost the same with the $198 of average middle-income countries, and reached to $426 in 2015, much higher than the $262 of middle-income countries, after a continued growth at an annual rate of approximately 23%, which was much faster than the growth rate of China's GDP and the global average health expenditure.

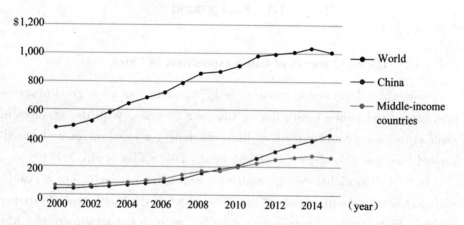

Figure 1-2　Health expenditure per capita of middle-income countries (2000-2015)

The rapidly rising of health care cost led to a heavy patient disease burden. From 1978 to 2002, the patient out-of-pocket payments grew from 20% to 60% of the total health expenditure, which was the highest patient out-of-pocket payment ratio in Asia. More than one-third of Chinese families were impoverished due to the expensive medical expending. (Hu et al., 2008; Yip & Hsiao, 2009) Figure 1-3 and Table 1-1 present the individual and household disease burden of rural and urban residents. From 2000 to 2013, the per capital health expenditure increased from 214.93 *yuan* to 1,274.44 *yuan* in rural areas, and from 812.95 *yuan* to 3,234.12 *yuan* in urban areas. From 2003 to 2011, the health spending as percentage of household income expenditure increased from 12.1% to 13.3% in rural areas, and from 9.3% to 11.9% in urban areas. (Meng et al., 2012)

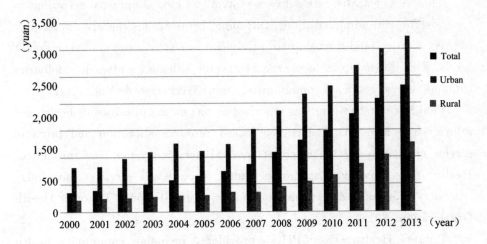

Figure 1-3   Per capita health expenditure (2000-2013)[1]

Table 1-1   Percentage of household income expenditure (2003-2011)

	2003	2008	2011	Average rate of change	
				2003-2008	2008-2011
Urban	9.3	10.6	11.9	1.4%	2.3%
Rural	12.1	12.6	13.3	0.9%	1.8%
Total	11.3	12.0	12.9	1.4%	2.3%

Using available healthcare resources in a more efficient and equitable way has become an important issue. In the first decade of 21st century, the greatest criticism of Chinese healthcare system was the poor access to health care, heavy disease burden (in Chinese as "kan bing nan", "kan bing gui") and huge inequity between urban and rural areas, which led to the waste and inefficiency of healthcare resource allocation. (Yip & Hsiao, 2009) To provide equal access to affordable basic health care, the new healthcare reform was introduced by the Chinese government in 2009. (Cheng, 2012)

---

① Data source: National Bureau of Statistics of China, National Health Service Survey.

1.1.2 The health care delivery system in China

The present health care delivery system in China is operated according to the government administration, including central, provincial, municipal, county, district, and township (in rural areas) or subdistrict (in urban areas) levels. Each township is in charge of several villages, and each subdistrict contains several residents communities. (Sun, Gregersen & Yuan, 2017)

Public hospital reform was launched as one of the priorities of healthcare reform since 2009. To reduce the biased resource allocation and promote service efficiency, the hierarchical medical service system was promoted. Healthcare service was categorized into three levels—tertiary hospitals, secondary hospitals and primary healthcare institutions. (World Health Organization, 2015)

Primary Health Care (PHC) providers, including community health centers in urban areas and township health centers and village clinics in rural areas, mainly undertake essential primary medical service and deliver comprehensive primary care and limited inpatient care for common diseases.

Secondary and tertiary hospitals carry out most outpatient and inpatient healthcare services. Tertiary hospitals, including most central, provincial and municipal hospitals, mainly provide emergency and critical care services for complex diseases and technical instruction to secondary hospitals. Secondary hospitals, including urban district hospitals and rural county hospitals, are responsible for basic medical care, emergency care, and technical instruction to physicians in primary hospitals.

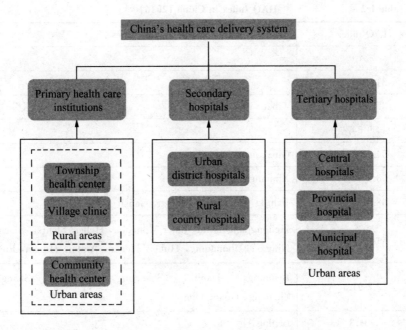

Figure 1-4   The three-tier level of China's health care delivery system

1.1.3   Poorer health access and quality performance in western China

Although more and more PHC providers in rural areas have been developed to provide basic healthcare service since the health reform, many backward regions still face the limited accessibility of health resources and inequity of health care performance. As reported in the Global Burden of Disease Study 2016, the Health Access and Quality (HAQ) index in China ranged from 91.5 in Beijing to 48.0 in Tibet, with a 43.5-point difference, showing large disparities in subnational levels, which is considered to be associated with factors including large variations in health expenditure per capita, physical access to health care facilities, provision of effective services across continuums of care, health care infrastructure and scale-up of medical technologies.

Table 1-2 shows the absolute differences of healthcare accessibility and quality among eastern, middle and western China.

Table 1-2 **HAQ Index in China (2016)** [①]

HAQ index	Provinces
<31.0	—
31.0-35.9	—
35.9-44.8	Tibet
44.9-54.7	—
54.7-63.2	Guizhou, Qinghai
63.2-68.9	Xinjiang, Yunnan
68.9-74.5	Jiangxi, Sichuan, Guangxi, Gansu
74.5-82.2	Heilongjiang, Jilin, Inner Mongolia, Hebei, Shanxi, Shaanxi, Ningxia, Chongqing, Hubei, Henan, Anhui, Hunan, Fujian
82.2-91.3	Liaoning, Tianjin, Shandong, Jiangsu, Shanghai, Zhejiang, Guangdong
>91.3	Beijing

The economic development of western China is still slower than other regions. At the end of 2014, the population of 11 western provinces was nearly 338.48 million, accounting for 1/4 of China's total population (1.37 billion), while the gross domestic product of western China represented only 19.2% of the nationally total amount. The GDP per capital of western China in 2014 was 37,487 *yuan*, less than 66,960 *yuan* of eastern China and 39,098 *yuan* of middle China.

Due to the gaps in terms of salary, living conditions and career prospects among different regions, most medical graduates tended to seek work opportunities in developed areas, secondary or tertiary healthcare facilities. (World Health Organization, 2015) Healthcare workforce shortage is observed in backward areas. In 2016, the number of licensed physicians per ten thousand residents in western China was 21.75, less than 26.09 in eastern China and 22.13 in middle China. While the number of registered nurses per 10 thousand residents in western China was only 24.00, less than 28.45 in eastern China.

---

① Data source: Global Burden of Disease Study (2016).

In western China, local county-level government budgets are relatively limited, the construction of local PHC institutions and health care infrastructure can only rely on the central and provincial budgets, while the service efficiency, health infrastructure construction and technology development variation may lead to the poorer health access and quality performance. The differences in economic and social development, health investment and demand for health services are also main factors that impact regional disparity in health human resources distribution. (World Health Organization, 2015) To reduce the inequality of health access and quality performance among different regions, except increasing capital investment and promoting universal health coverage, more efforts are still needed to analyze health demand of local residents, and further improve the resource allocation efficiency.

1.1.4 Patient perception of healthcare service and resource allocation efficiency

Consumption behavior is a process. Consumers' perception of quality and value is considered as a crucial determinant of purchase behavior and product choice. Consumers' perceived quality can be conceptualized as consumer's judgment about the overall excellence or superiority of a product/service, while the perceived value is defined as the consumer's assessment of the utility of perceived benefits and sacrifices (cost). Consumers' perception presents individual preference and results in behavioral intention, being reflected in consumer decision process, that is, before, during, and after the purchase. (Choi et al., 2004; Zeithaml, 1988)

Correspondingly, in health care, consumer (patient) perception is a reflection of patient demand and preference of healthcare service, which is directly associated with quality and value of care service. Since the patient value assessment is also influenced by perceived service quality, healthcare service quality has direct impact on the patient decision process, which could be understood through the patient health seeking behavior and satisfaction of healthcare service.(Choi et al., 2004; Zeithaml, 1988)

Therefore, patient perception of healthcare service reveals patient demand. It is an important indicator for measuring the service performance, plays crucial role in promoting clinical outcomes and hospital competitiveness, and is beneficial in improving resource utilization efficiency and increasing the effectiveness of healthcare system. Investigating patient perception of health care service is essential to both care providers and payers.

1.1.5 Existing studies about outpatient perception of health care service in China

Some researchers had explored the patient health-seeking behaviors and the choice of care providers in China, mostly from urban areas with single-center evidence, mainly about elder residents and chronic patients, indicating that patients' characteristics including socioeconomic status, education level, medical insurance coverage, marriage status, residence and illness severity were associated with patients' choice of care provider, and external factors including the hospital distance, service attitude, doctors' and nurses' professional skills, drug availability and medical cost were also dominant reasons.

Chinese outpatient satisfaction and associated factors had also been discussed, mostly in developed provinces or tertiary hospitals, with descriptive analysis and satisfaction ratings survey as most common methods. Factors including hospital environment, medical facility, service attitude, patients' involvement in decision making, doctors' and nurses' proficient skills, effective communication between patients and doctors, disease severity, medical cost, waiting time and service time were proved to be associated with Chinese outpatients' satisfaction in advanced areas or tertiary hospitals.

1.2　Research gaps

Outpatient perception analysis including outpatient health seeking behavior and satisfaction of healthcare service is an important indicator for evaluating the service quality, which should be essential for both healthcare service payers and providers. Therefore, it is necessary to conduct the patient perception analysis in rural western China, to improve care efficiency, and to further promote the accessibility and quality of health care service in backward areas.

According to Grossman's concept of demand for health, patients' demands for medical services are associated with demographic characteristics and socio-economic conditions, so patients' perception in backward areas should be measured in a different way from developed areas. Since no questionnaire study was processed to study the outpatient satisfaction and the choice of care providers, with a large-sample evidence from different backward provinces, considering the local residents' demographic characteristics, socio-economic status and heavier economic burden, a region-specific questionnaire should be performed to study the outpatient perception of health care service performance in rural western China.

1.3 Research questions and hypotheses

Patient perception of healthcare service could be adopted to reveal patient demands, and to evaluate the performance of service quality, accessibility and efficiency, which can be explained by patient satisfaction and choice of care providers. Although previous studies have explored the Chinese outpatient satisfaction and relevant factors in developed areas and tertiary hospitals, similar studies have been conducted to investigate the patient perception of outpatient service in backward areas. Consequently, the main objective of this study was to conduct a region-specific questionnaire survey for the outpatient perception of health care service performance in rural western China, including the satisfaction of primary outpatient service and patient choice of care providers, while policy recommendations will also be concluded to improve the efficiency of resource allocation and reduce the huge inequity between urban and rural areas. The research questions and hypotheses are listed as below:

Question 1: What is outpatients' first choice of health care providers for common illness in rural western China?

Hypothesis 1: Different outpatients would choose different healthcare facilities. Since most basic medical services are delivered by PHC providers, township health centers or village clinics should be the most common options in rural western China.

Question 2: Are there any internal factors significantly associated with outpatients' choices of care providers, and what are these factors?

Hypothesis 2: According to previous evidence, internal factors including outpatient demographic characteristics, disease severity, medical coverage should have significant impact on the choices of care providers.

Question 3: Are there any external factors significantly associated with outpatients' choices of care providers, and what are these factors?

Hypothesis 3: As reported in existing references, hospital location, service attitude, doctors' and nurses' professional skills, drug supply and medical cost would be main external factors significantly associated with outpatients' choices of care provider.

Question 4: How satisfied are outpatients with the medical service in rural western China?

Hypothesis 4: Due to the limited accessibility and poorer healthcare service performance, outpatients' satisfaction in rural western China would be relatively lower than that in developed areas and tertiary hospitals.

Question 5: Are there any factors significantly associated with outpatients' satisfaction of medical service in rural western China, and what are these factors?

Hypothesis 5: Factors including outpatient demographic characteristics, medical coverage and disease severity should be significantly associated with outpatients' satisfaction.

1.4 Potential contribution

Firstly, from the perspective of patients, the outpatient satisfaction and the choice of health care providers could interpret outpatient demands to care providers and payers and patient perception analysis would be an important approach to improving health care service quality. Mean while the results of this study could be used to improve resident health status, reduce individual and household disease burden and promote healthcare accessibility in backward areas.

Secondly, for healthcare service providers, understanding patient demands could increase the efficiency of service. Outpatients' perception of healthcare service in rural western China could illustrate outpatient preference and health seeking behavior, which would help to set an appropriate measurement for local healthcare service performance, and further promote clinical outcomes and hospital competitiveness of healthcare facilities in rural western China.

Thirdly, patients' perception of health care outpatient service in rural western China would indicate outpatients' demands and preference, enhance hospital quality and efficiency of service and encourage the rational utilization of healthcare resources. Therefore, for policy makers and healthcare service payers, the patient perception analysis in rural western China could play a crucial part in cutting improper expenditure, reducing inequity in health care between urban and rural areas, and promoting the universal access to basic health care.

1.5 Research approach and organization

The flow chart in Figure 1-5 shows the research approach of part I of this book.

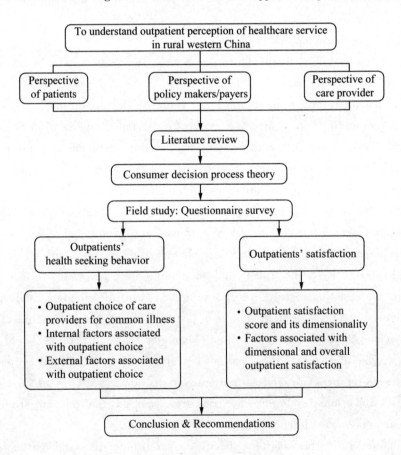

Figure 1-5 Research approach

This research was performed from the perspective of patients, policy makers/health payers and health care providers (health care facilities). Literature and document review was conducted to describe China's current health system, address the concept for patient perception and clarify the related theories, while relevant studies were also screened to extract adaptive information for questionnaire development. The main framework of the field study was constructed based on the Consumer Decision Process Theory, and a questionnaire survey was conducted to collect information about outpatient choice of care providers and outpatient satisfaction in rural western China. Descriptive analysis and statistical analysis were processed to investigate outpatients' choices of care providers, satisfaction degree and relevant factors. Finally, conclusion and recommendations were provided based on the results of data analysis.

There are six chapters as below:

Chapter 1: This chapter introduces the background of this research, describes the rapid growth of health expenditure and hierarchical medical system in China, and puts forward the issue of the poorer performance of health accessibility and quality in western China. Patient perception of health care service is essential for understanding patients' demands and promoting care efficiency. Although previous reports have discussed patient seeking behavior and satisfaction, none researches have been conducted in rural western China, covering several provinces. The research gap still exists, based on which research questions and hypotheses are formulated. The research approach and potential contribution are also clarified in this chapter.

Chapter 2: Relevant studies and documents were reviewed, with related theories and existing research results summarized in this chapter. Evolvement of Chinese health care system and medical insurance schemes are included, and the concepts of patient perception and Consumer Decision Process Theory are clarified. Existing studies about patient perception are screened, the outpatient health seeking behavior and outpatient satisfaction researches in developed countries and some developing countries are discussed, and relevant studies in China are taken as reference for questionnaire design.

Chapter 3: In this chapter, specific research objectives and methodology are illustrated. Five specific research objectives are clarified, and the research design of each specific objective and questionnaire development are addressed. Data collection procedure, data sampling and statistics methods are also listed in Chapter 3.

Chapter 4: The statistical results of questionnaire of outpatients' choice of care providers in rural western China are interpreted in Chapter 4, including descriptive findings of outpatients' choice and respondents' characteristics. Internal factors and external factors associated with outpatients' health seeking behavior are also addressed through results of multinomial logistics regression and Chi-square analysis.

Chapter 5: The results of the questionnaire are explained in this chapter. Participant characteristics and outpatient satisfaction item scores are presented through descriptive analysis. The result of Exploratory Factor Analysis (EFA) addresses the structural dimensionality of overall outpatient satisfaction. Patient characteristics associated with overall and dimensional satisfaction are demonstrated with results of stepwise multilinear regression.

Chapter 6: This chapter concludes the whole dissertation, and provides recommendations for policy makers, health care payers and providers. In the meantime, limitations of this research and prospects of future work are also illustrated in this chapter.

Chapter 2　Literature review

2.1　Health care system in China

2.1.1　Evolvement of health care system in China

China's health care delivery system and medical insurance scheme evolved with the healthcare service system. There are 4 phases according to recent reports.

During the first phase (1949-1983), China started the government-owned health institutions and funded almost all medical spending of government staff and enterprise employees in urban areas. The Rural Cooperative Medical System (RCMS) was established in rural areas, and public-subsidized barefoot doctors were main medical workers in village level. Health status of Chinese resident have been significantly improved since the establishment of People's Republic of China (PRC). (Sun et al., 2017)

The second phase (1984-2002) began after China's economic reform and opening-up in the late 1970s. The village-based agricultural collective farming system was replaced by the new household-responsibility system, since when the RCMS lost its institutional basis and collapsed in a short time. In 1980s, many state-owned enterprises went bankrupt. Without public medical coverage and private insurance industry, the free-market health care system means the majority of population had no medical insurance. In 1998, only 38% of urban residents were covered by any kind of medical insurance, and the percentage of insured resident in rural areas was only 7% in 1999. By the late 1990s, limited access to health care and heavy disease burden aroused great public discontents. At the end of 1998, the Chinese Government launched the Urban Employee Basic Medical Insurance (UEBMI), covering enterprise employees and retirees in urban areas.

In the third phase (2003-2008), further reform on the health insurance scheme was processed. In 2003, Chinese government issued the New Rural Cooperative Medical Scheme (NRCMS), which covers rural residents. In 2008, the Urban Residents Basic Medical Insurance (URBMI) was introduced, which covers urban citizens including children, students, elderly people, and unemployed people. Only one inpatient expenditure was reimbursement at the early stage. (Sun et al., 2017)

In the fourth phase (from 2009 to now), Chinese government concluded that reform of both insurance and the health care delivery systems was necessary to promote the accessibility and equity of healthcare service. A more comprehensive health care reform has been initiated since 2009, mainly including five priorities: 1) accelerating the development of basic medical security system; 2) establishing the national essential medicine system; 3) promoting primary healthcare service; 4) strengthening the equity of basic public healthcare service, and 5) initiating the pilot projects in public hospital reform.

A new five-year road-map for the reform of health sector was introduced according to the National Planning Guideline for the Healthcare Service System (2015-2020). The recent emphases include infrastructure development, cost reducing and insurance coverage broadening, and investment on new areas. (General Office of the State Council of the People's Republic of China, 2015a) Improving the geographic accessibility in high demand regions such as western China and rural areas, promoting health resource allocation, relieving the problem in the doctor-patient relationship are also mentioned in the Notice on Few Key Points on the Healthcare System Reform in 2018. (General Office of the State Council of the People's Republic of China, 2018) Table 2-1 demonstrates the evolution of health care system in China.

Table 2-1　　　　　**The evolution of China's health care system**

Year	Key events
1949	The Peoples' Republic of China was founded.
the 1950s	Government-funded Insurance System was launched as a public insurance program for government and enterprise employees. The Rural Cooperative Medical System (RCMS) was established at the village level.
the late 1970s	Economic reform and opening-up initiated, the planned economy collapsed, and the village-based agricultural collective farming system was replaced by the new household-responsibility system in rural areas.
the 1980s	The RCMS lost its institutional basis and collapsed.
the 1990s	The majority of urban residents and employees lost health insurance.
1998	Urban Employee Basic Medical Insurance (UEBMI) was launched, which covers enterprise employees and retirees in urban areas.
2003	New Rural Cooperative Medical Scheme (NRCMS) was implemented nation-wide in rural areas.
2008	The Urban Residents Basic Medical Insurance (URBMI) was introduced, which covers urban citizens including children, students, elderly people, and unemployed people.
since 2009	The new health care reform has been promoting the accessibility and equity of healthcare service.

2.1.2　Health coverage in China

China's current health insurance system mainly consists of three health insurance schemes, including the Urban Employee Basic Medical Insurance (UEBMI), the Urban Residents Basic Medical Insurance (URBMI) and the New Rural Cooperative Medical Scheme (NRCMS).

In the middle 1980s and the early 1990s, the majority of urban workers lost health insurance during the economic transition. The UEBMI was initiated in 1994 and formally launched in 1998 as a replacement of previous urban insurance system. The UEBMI is a compulsory basic medical insurance covering employees and retirees of state-owned and private enterprise in urban areas, funded by employers and employees. The reimbursement rate of inpatient care in UEBMI is 80%, while the outpatient payment rate varied in different provinces. In 2016, 295 million of urban employees and retirees were covered by the UEBMI, and the enrollment rate was higher than 95%.

In 2003, after the collapse of planned economy and Rural Cooperative Medical System (RCMS), to promote national health care equity and balance social development between urban and rural areas, the NRCMS was proposed under the strategy of building a "harmonious society" as a voluntary basic health insurance scheme covering rural residents. The NRCMS is mostly funded by government subsidies, with a small proportion contributed by individual. At the beginning, the NRCMS program only payed for inpatient care. Since 2009, outpatient care has been covered after that the division of premium pooled into outpatient funds and inpatient funds. In addition, the annual payment premium is six-times income of local farmers. By 2016, 275 million of rural residents have been involved in the NRCMS, which means the enrollment rate has reached to 99% of total rural population. (Liang & Langenbrunner, 2013; Sun et al., 2017)

The urban unemployed residents, students and children are the last group to be covered by the public health insurance scheme. Funded by government and individual, the URBMI project was piloted in 2007 and formally launched in 2008, which is a voluntary basic health care insurance covering urban citizens including children, students, seniors, disabled, and unemployed people. In the early stage, the URBMI covered only inpatient care. Since 2009, outpatient care has been included. And the reimbursement rate has reached to 70% for inpatients and 50% for outpatients in 2014. (General Office of the State Council of the People's Republic of China, 2015b) The annual reimbursement premium of URBMI is six-times disposable income of local residents. In 2016, 453 million of enrollees were covered by URBMI, and the enrollment rate was higher than 95%. (Liang & Langenbrunner, 2013; Sun et al., 2017)

By the end of 2016, more than 1.3 billion Chinese were covered by basic health insurance system, and the overall coverage rate was higher than 95%, which marks the achievement of universal health coverage in China. (State Council Information Office of the People's Republic of China, 2017)

Table 2-2 summarizes the characteristics of China's current health insurance system.

Table 2-2   **Summary of China's health insurance system**[①]

	UEBMI	URBMI	NRCMS
Target population	Urban employees and retirees	Urban residents, including children, student, the unemployed and the disabled	Urban residents, including children, student, the unemployed and the disabled
Type of enrollment	Compulsory	Voluntary	Voluntary
Source of funding	Employers and employees	Government and individual	Government and individual
Annual reimbursement premium	Six-times average wage of employees in cities	Six-times average disposable income of local residents	Six-times average income of local farmers
Facts in 2016			
Number of enrollees (million)	295	453	670
Enrollment rate (%)	>95%	>95%	99%
Proportion of total population (%)	21	32	48
Reimbursement for inpatient care (%)	80	70	70

---

① Data source: Yearbook of National Health and Family Planning Commission of PRC.

2.2 Patient perception of health care service

2.2.1 Concept of consumer perception

Consumer behavior is a process in which individuals or groups select, purchase, use, or dispose of products, service, ideas, or experience to satisfy needs and desires. A consumer's purchase behavior is influenced by cultural, social, and personal factors. There are three stages in the consumption process, including pre-purchase stage, purchase stage and post-purchase stage, during which customers' requirements, expectations, perceptions, satisfaction, and loyalty would influence the purchase decision. (Kotler et al., 2016; Solomon et al., 2014)

In marketing, consumer perception is more important than reality because consumer perception of quality and value is considered to be dominant factors associated with actual purchase behavior. Consumer's perceived quality suggests consumer's experience about the overall excellence or superiority of the product/service, while the perceived value demonstrates the consumer's evaluation of the utility of perceived benefits and sacrifices (cost) of the product/service. Consumer perception presents individual preference and results in behavioral intention, being reflected before, during, and after the purchase behavior process.

2.2.2 Patient perception of health care service

Consumer's behaviors in medical process are changing from passive to aggressive. In the relationship of patients and hospitals, patients should be considered as consumers of medical service in the medical care market, while health facilities are major service providers. (Lee, Shih & Chung, 2008) Like other product purchase process, health care service consuming is also one kind of consumer behavior. Patient perceived quality and value will have direct impact on patient satisfaction, and further influence patient behavior intentions and health-seeking decision. Since patient value perception is influenced by health care service quality, patient experience of health care summarized by patient decision behavior process is becoming a main measurement of health care quality performance.(Choi et al., 2004)

According to existing studies, defining a proper measurement of health care quality contributes to improving the efficiency of health care resource allocation and reducing the uneven care between developed and backward areas. In US hospitals, patient experiences of care are investigated through the Hospital Consumer Assessment of Healthcare Providers and Systems (HCAHPS) survey, to improve the performance of care and encourage consumers to make informed health care choices. (Isaac, Zaslavsky, Cleary & Landon, 2010; Jha, Orav, Zheng & Epstein, 2008)

Patient experiences with health care are related with care service quality, which also influences patient purchase decision. Patient perception of healthcare service suggests patient demand, plays an important role in promoting clinical outcomes and hospital competitiveness, and is beneficial in improving resource utilization efficiency and increasing the effectiveness of healthcare system. Therefore, exploring patient perception is necessary to both health care providers and payers.

In this study, patient decision process is explored to understand the sources and consequences of patient perception of health care service.

2.3 Consumer decision process theory

2.3.1 Concept of consumer decision process

Consumer decision is a complicated synthesis of process used by consumers regarding market transactions before, during, and after the purchase of a product or service. (Blackwell, Miniard & Engel, 2006) A consumer's buying decision includes the psychological construct, the judgement of what the consumer needs or wants, the awareness of various product/service choices, the information-gathering activity, and the evaluation of alternatives. (Schiffman & Wisenblit, 2018) The buying decision starts before the actual purchase behavior, and has consequences long afterward. The purchase behavior is never the end of the decision process. (Howard & Sheth, 1969; Kotler et al., 2016)

Table 2-3 presents a list of some key questions about consumer decision that marketers should ask, in terms of who, what, when, where, how, and why.(Kotler et al., 2016)

Table 2-3	Understanding the consumer decision
Who does buy the product/service?	
Who does make the decision to buy the product/service?	
Who does influence the decision to buy the product/service?	
How is the buying decision made? Who assumes what role?	
What does the consumer buy? What needs must be satisfied? What wants are fulfilled?	
Why do consumers buy a particular brand? What benefits do they seek?	
Where do they go or look to buy the product or service? Online and/or offline?	
When do they buy? Any seasonality factors? Any time of a day/week/month?	
How is our product or service perceived by customers?	
What are customers' attitudes toward our products/service?	
What social factors might influence the purchase decision?	
Do customers' lifestyles influence their decisions?	
How do personal, demographic, or economic factors influence the purchase decision?	

A consumer's buying decision behavior is influenced by cultural, social, and personal factors (Solomon et al., 2014), while Grossman (1972) proposed in the concept of health demand that patient demand is associated with demographic characteristics and socio-economic status, indicating that patient perception is also associated with external factors and internal factors.

2.3.2 Different types of consumer decision process

According to existing theories of classification, consumer decision behaviors are classified into different types. Assael (1984) proposed four types of consumer decision making process according to the degree of consumer involvement with the product and the brand difference (see Table 2-4). (Assael, 1984) Schiffman (2018) analyzed consumer decision behavior based on the degree of information research before consumers evaluate and choose a product/service, and consumer decision behaviors are divided into extensive problem solving, limited problem solving and routinized problem solving (see Table 2-5). (Schiffman & Wisenblit, 2018)

Table 2-4 **Assael's consumer behavior classification**

	High consumer involvement	Low consumer involvement
Significant differences between bands	Complex buying behavior	Variety seeking behavior
Few differences between brands	Dissonance-reducing buying behavior	Habitual buying behavior

Table 2-5 **Schiffman's consumer decision behavior classification**

	Characteristics
Extensive problem solving	Consumers have no established criterion, and need extensive information search and evaluation of alternatives, typically when making expensive purchases, e.g. cars, diamonds.
Limited problem solving	Consumers have established the basic criteria, but need more information to decide among alternatives, and it often occurs when consumers make familiar purchases, e.g. new laptop.
Routinized response behavior	Consumers have experience with the product category and alternatives, and it often occurs when consumers make habitual purchases.

In this study, three types of consumer decision making process are proposed, according to the different sequence of steps involving consumers' thinking, feeling, and eventually doing, as Michael Solomon stated in the *Consumer behavior*: *buying, having and being*.

Cognitive decision making is a rational process in which consumers integrate information about the product/service, weigh the strength and shortage of each alternative, and arrive at the most satisfactory decision. It is an outcome of a series of stages that results in the selection of a product/service among competing options. Deliberate, rational and sequential thinking is the key point that determines cognitive decision approach, which is especially relevant to activities concerned with financial planning and choices that impact consumers' quality of life. (Solomon et al., 2014)

Habitual decision making is more like a routine process without logical purposes, which is made with certain assumptions rather than collecting information about alternatives. Although automatic choices based on little or no conscious effort may lead to mental accounting biases, habitual decision making is quite an efficient way in some cases, for example, buying low-cost products in supermarket. (Solomon et al., 2014)

Affective decision making is rather an emotional response than a rational approach, which is always an instantaneous reaction relevant with mood or emotion. Consumers tend to make affective decisions to satisfy emotional needs. (Solomon et al., 2014)

Purchasing behavior for health care is directly associated with consumers' quality of life, so the consumer decision in the health care market is a cognitive decision process.

2.3.3 Stages of consumer decision process

The consumer decision process usually consists of five stages: problem/need recognition, information search, evaluation of alternatives, purchase decision, and post-purchase behavior, of which the first three stages are before the actual purchase, and the last one is after the purchase. (Kotler et al., 2016; Solomon et al., 2014)

Problem/need recognition is the very first stage of buying decision process. When the consumer recognizes a problem or need triggered by internal or external stimuli, e.g. hunger, illness and admiration of a friend's new car, it rises and becomes a drive to seek for a specific product or service to solve the problem or satisfy the need. (Kotler et al., 2016; Solomon et al., 2014) During the health care approach, patients' illness recognition is the direct reason that arouses the health seeking behavior.

Once a consumer recognizes a problem/need, he/she would like to solve/satisfy it. The consumer considers that each product/service is a bundle of attributes with varying abilities to deliver the benefits. Information search is the process that the consumer studies the environment for adaptive data to evaluate the benefits behind each attribute and make the appropriate decision.

(Solomon et al., 2014) And the major information sources fall into 4 groups: personal (family, friends), public (social media), commercial (ads, salespersons) and experiential (tester, examining).(Kotler et al., 2016) As previously reported, in the approach of medical care, before visiting the hospital, patient would evaluate the relevant external factors, such as hospital distance, waiting time, medical charge, doctors' professional skills and so on.

After the information gathering, multiple products/service are revealed, the consumer would compare the appropriateness of each searched alternative and make the judgement. Alternatively, evaluation may occur continuously throughout the entire consumer decision process. (Kotler et al., 2016) Before choosing the care provider, except external information, internal factors such as patient socio-economic status, insurance coverage rate and disease severity are also proved to be significant associations. The evaluation on the alternative hospitals would be conducted based on both the external and internal factors.

Once all attributes of alternatives have been evaluated, the consumer forms the preference among alternative options and executes the buying intention. In this stage, patients choose the care providers based on the evaluation of hospitals and individual characteristics. (Kotler et al., 2016)

Following the purchase and after experiencing the product/service, the consumer would get to the final stage, namely post-purchase behavior. In this stage, the consumer compares expectations and the perceived performance of the purchased product/service, and the results will influence the decision process for similar purchase in the future. Satisfied consumers tend to purchase the same product/service again, while the unsatisfied consumers will refuse to purchase the same product/service next time. (Kotler et al., 2016) To ensure the choice of appropriate care providers and promote efficiency of resource utilization, understanding patient satisfaction after the health care is critical for not only patients, but also health care providers and payers.

Figure 2-1 depicts the five stages of patient decision process when patients choose the health care providers.

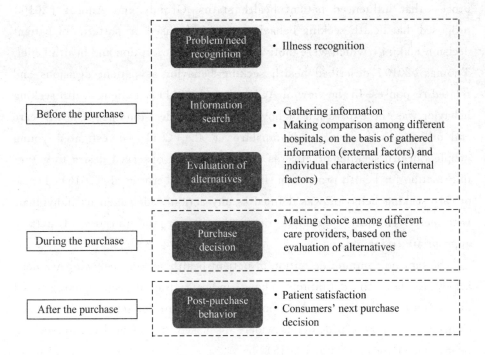

Figure 2-1　Stages of consumer decision process

In this study, outpatient health seeking behavior in Stage 4 and post-purchase satisfaction in Stage 5 are analyzed to evaluate outpatient perceived care performance, and associated factors in the stage 2 and stage 3 are explored to understand the source of outpatient perception.

2.4　Patient choice of care provider

2.4.1　Concept of health seeking behavior

According to Ahmed (2000), health seeking behavior refers to a sequence of remedial action that individuals undertake to rectify perceived ill-health. The concepts of health seeking behavior evolved with time, based as reviewed literature, several varied definitions of health seeking behavior were concluded. Babar and Hatcher (2004) defined patient health seeking behavior as making decisions about choices of health facilities. Jackson et al. (2004) pointed out that patient health seeking behavior was an decision-making process that influenced patient health status. Grundy and Annear (2010) proposed that health seeking behavior analysis focused on patterns of patient decision-making, which were motivated by illness perception and health belief. Thomas (2010) described health seeking behavior as patient decisions and related responses. In the view of Agarwal et al. (2011), patient health seeking behavior was the expression of how people made decisions about health care and utilization of services. Hampshire et al. (2011) investigated young people's health seeking practice as an expressed or observed desire to gather information for health promotion. In the view of Oberoi et al. (2016), health or care seeking behavior was defined as any action undertaken by individuals with perceived health problem or to be ill for the purpose of getting appropriate treatment.

So far, no common definition of patient health seeking behavior has been achieved, but all definitions above indicate the decision-making-based dimension of health seeking behavior concept. Patient decision to seek care and choice of health care provider is widely discussed among health care seeking behaviors. (Poortaghi et al., 2015)

2.4.2 Theories of patient health seeking behavior

A variety of widely used theories and models of health seeking behavior have been developed. Glanz, Rimer and Viswanath introduced four contemporary theories of individual health-related behavior in *Health behavior and health education: theory, research, and practice* (2008), including The Health Belief Model (HBM), the Theory of Reasoned Action (TRA) and the Theory of Planned Behavior (TPB), the Transtheoretical Model (TTM)/ Stage of Change (SOC) and the Precaution Adoption Process Model (PAPM).

The Health Belief Model (HBM) was developed initially in the 1950s by social psychologists in the U.S. Public Health Service, to explain changes and maintenance of patient health-related behaviors, and was gradually evolved to support the interventions to change health behavior. HBM is a cognitively based model, considering no emotional components, and it contains several concepts that predict why people will take action to prevent, to screen for, or to control illness conditions. Only internal factors such as demographic information, socio-economic status and knowledge are considered to be associated with individual beliefs. And no external factor is included in HBM. Figure 2-2 presents the construct of HBM. (Hochbaum, 1958)

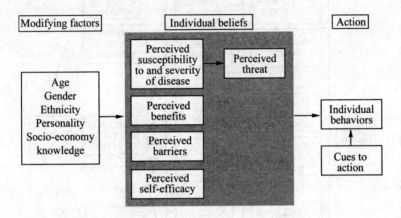

Figure 2-2   Construct of the health belief model

In the view of Fishbein (1967), the Theory of Reasoned Action (TRA) was developed to understand relationships among attitudes, intentions, and behaviors. TRA assumes that the critical predictor of behavior is the behavioral intention, which is determined by attitude towards the behavior and social normative perceptions, while the Theory of Planned Behavior (TPB) adds perceived control over behavior intention. The Integrated Behavioral Model (IBM) was proposed later, combining constructs from TRA, TPB and components from other behavior theories. Figure 2-3 shows the construct of IBM.

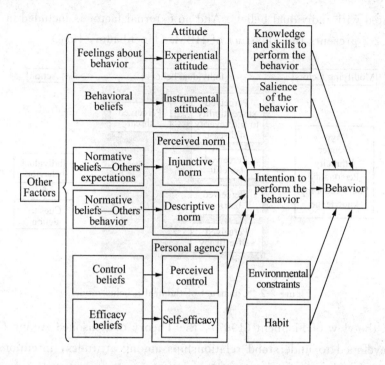

Figure 2-3　Constructs of the integrated behavioral model

The Transtheoretical Model (TTM) uses stages of change to integrate processes and principles of change across major theories of intervention, and it is also known as Stage of Change (SOC). And TTM interventions can be performed in return to change patient health behaviors. A series of six stages of change (precontemplation, contemplation, preparation, action, maintenance and termination), ten processes of change (consciousness raising, dramatic relief, self-reevaluation, environmental reevaluation, self-liberation, helping relationships, counterconditioning, reinforcement management, stimulus control and social liberation), decision balance and self-efficacy construct TTM.

The Precaution Adoption Process Model (PAPM) was initially stimulated by Irving Janis and Leon Mann (1977). Nowadays, PAPM seeks to identify all the stages involved when people perform health-protective behaviors and to investigate the factors that lead people to move from one stage to the next. (Glanz, Rimer & Viswanath, 2008; Janis & Mann, 1979)

In recent decades, HBM has become one of the most frequently used conceptual frameworks to analyze and describe health-related behavior, determining relationships between individual health beliefs and health behaviors.

2.4.3   Existing studies about patient choice of health care provider

Most existing studies about patient choice of health care providers referred to more than one model as the theoretical basis. In most studies, not only individual factors, but also external influences such as hospital facility, doctors' professional skills, staff attitude, medical charge were investigated as the resources of patient perception and behavioral intentions.

Previous studies have revealed that patients' health care seeking behavior was influenced by a combination of patient and provider characteristics, including patients' age, education level, income, providers' location, service quality and effective patient-doctor communications. (Victoor et al., 2012) In developed countries, provider characteristics were frequently discussed. As stated by Merks et al. (2004), the most frequently reported factors that influenced patient choice in UK were professional and high quality of service, then location and good advice received from care providers. According to Birk, Gut and Henriksen (2011), outpatients from Denmark considered the distance was the most critical reason determining the choice of hospital, followed by the GP's recommendations, waiting time, and the patient's previous perception with the hospital. In United States, patients chose primary care provider based on physicians' technical skills rather than interpersonal quality. (Fung et al., 2005) Several developing countries, such as India, Eritrea, Vietnam and Gnana, have also investigated patient health seeking behavior, proving that patients' health-seeking behavior was significantly influenced by disease severity and patient demographic characteristics, especially economic status and education level. Availability of essential drugs, distance, provider reputation, doctors' professional skills, medical charges and patient residence were also considered as main factors when patient from rural areas select the primary healthcare provider.

In traditional Chinese doctor-patient relationship, patients were not encouraged to actively engage in the caregiving process. Patient involvement and participation in healthcare decisions were only recently promoted since

1990s, to improve the health care efficiency and patient adherence. (W. Zhang et al., 2014) In recent years, some researchers have explored patient health-seeking behavior, mostly from urban areas with single-center evidence, mainly about elder residents and chronic patients, indicating that patients' characteristics such as individual socioeconomic status, education level, medical insurance coverage, marriage status, residence and illness severity are associated with patients' choice of care provider, while external factors including the hospital distance, service attitude, doctors' and nurses' professional skills, drug availability and medical cost are also dominant reasons.

2.5 Patient satisfaction

2.5.1 Concept of patient satisfaction

Consumer satisfaction/dissatisfaction presents the overall attitude a person has about a product/service after it has been purchased. (Kotler et al., 2016) There is no commonly accepted definition of consumer satisfaction, and significant differences are contained in the reviewed literature. A basic definitional inconsistency is about whether the satisfaction is an evaluation process or an outcome/response of the evaluation process. (Yi, 1990)

Some researchers defined the satisfaction as an evaluation process. An often-cited definition was provided by Hunt Institute and Foundation (1977), defining consumer satisfaction with a product/service as the favorableness of the individual's subjective evaluation of the various outcomes and experiences associated with purchasing it or using it. And a similar opinion was given by Oliver (1981), considering consumer satisfaction as an evaluation of the surprise inherent in a product/service acquisition and/or purchase experience.

In marketing, consumer satisfaction is always conceptualized as an omnibus noun representing most events occurring after a customer makes a purchase. Therefore, most definitions have favored the notion of consumer satisfaction as an outcome/response to an evaluation process. According to Locke (1969), Westbrook (1980) and Woodruff et al. (1983), consumer satisfaction is described as an emotion response from appraisals (including disconfirmation, perceived performance, etc.) of a set of experiences. More precisely, consumer satisfaction reflects a person's judgment of the perceived performance of a purchased product/service in relationship to expectations. If performance falls short of expectations, the consumer is dissatisfied. If it matches expectations, the consumer is satisfied.(Kotler et al., 2016)

Most patient satisfaction formulations are developed from both the marketing and health care fields. In this study, patient satisfaction refers to consumer evaluation with health care service performance after purchasing and experiencing the care. Pasco (1983) defined patient satisfaction as "recipient's reaction to salient aspects of the context, process and result of their service experience". While Swan et al. (1985) considered patient satisfaction as an emotional response to the experience of hospitalization, but it is a cognitive process of comparing results to standards. Similarly, Eriksen (1995) identified patient satisfaction as a rating of evaluation of a provider or service based on a comparison of the patient's subjective standards to care received, presenting a positive emotional response to the comparison. According to Hills and Kitchen (2007), patient satisfaction was described as a sense of contentedness, achievement or fulfillment that results from meeting patients' needs and expectations with respect to specific and general aspects of health care.

All the definitions above have three characteristics in common: 1) patient satisfaction is an emotional or affective evaluation of the care service/provider based on cognitive processes which were influenced by expectations; 2) patient satisfaction is a congruence of expectations and actual experiences of the health care service; 3) patient satisfaction is an overall evaluation of different aspects of the care service. (Batbaatar et al., 2015)

2.5.2　Theories of patient satisfaction

Most of patient satisfaction theories were published in the 1980s, and summarized again in recent years. There are five key theories listed below:

Discrepancy and transgression theory of Fox and Storm (1981) advocated that patient satisfaction was associated with patients' healthcare orientations and conditions of care provider. That is, if orientations and conditions were congruent, patients were satisfied, and if not, patients were dissatisfied.

Expectancy-value theory of Linder-Pelz (1982) proposed that patient satisfaction was mediated by individual beliefs and values about care as well as prior expectations about care. Then the theory was developed by Pascoe (1983), emphasizing the influence of expectations on satisfaction, while Strasser (1993) established a six-factor psychological model: cognitive and affective perception formation; multidimensional construct; dynamic process; attitudinal response; iterative; and ameliorated by individual difference.

Determinants and components theory of Ware et al. (1983) suggested that patient satisfaction was a function of patients' subjective responses to experienced care mediated by personal preferences and expectations.

Multiple model theory of Fitzpatrick and Hopkins (1983) indicated that patient expectation was a reflection of the health goals of patients, which were socially mediated, demonstrating the extent to which illness and health care violated the patient sense of self.

Health care quality theory of Donabedian (1980) propounded that satisfaction was the principal outcome of the interpersonal process of care. He argued that the expression of satisfaction or dissatisfaction is the patient's judgement on the quality of care in all its aspects, but particularly in relation to the interpersonal component of care.

2.5.3 Measurement of patient satisfaction

Patient satisfaction has become an important endpoint in clinical outcomes research and benchmarking of healthcare services, influenced by cultural, sociodemographic, cognitive and affective components. (Aharony & Strasser, 1993; Heidegger, Saal & Nuebling, 2006) There are many different methods for assessing patient satisfaction with health care and various surveys have been published. Some methods are based on observing consumers, and others are on directly approaching consumers to elicit evaluations. Questionnaire is one of the most popular means of collecting patient evaluations. One of the most frequently used approach in satisfaction studies is the Likert scale, where respondents are required to rate aspects of care service or state the extent to which they agree/disagree with predetermined statements, and scores can be summoned to assess each item. Other possible scaling techniques include verbal frequency scales, rankings, linear numerical scales, semantic scales and adjective checklists. (Crow et al., 2002)

The majority of patient satisfaction studies employed self-designed questionnaires based on a review of existing scales. (Gill & White, 2009) Hulka et al. (1970) initialized the first measurement instrument of patient satisfaction in the healthcare area, with the Satisfaction with Physician and Primary Care Scale (SPPCS). Then Ware and Snyder (1975) developed the Patient Satisfaction Questionnaire (PSQ), assisting with the planning, administration and evaluation of health service delivery programs. At the end of the 1970s, the Client Satisfaction Questionnaire (CSQ) was designed by Larsen et al. (1979), assessing general patient satisfaction with health care services, and was replaced by the Patient Satisfaction Scale (PSS) in 1984. Sometimes the measurement of patient satisfaction varies due to the research assumptions. The Quality of Care from the Patient's Perspective (QCPP) has often been measured as patient satisfaction. And the Patient Judgment of Hospital Quality (PJHQ) was also designed to represent patient view. (Gill & White, 2009; Meterko et al., 1990)

In recent decades, numerous instruments have been developed, but most of which validation and reliability are still remained to be reported. (Gill & White, 2009)

2.5.4 Existing studies about patient satisfaction

Most patient satisfaction studies were conducted in US and European countries, suggesting patients in flourishing regions tend to evaluate the quality of health care service based on waiting time, medical staffs' proficiency, hospital environment and participation in the medical decision making. There are several recent patient assessment studies, which have been conducted in developing countries, including India, Thailand, Tanzania and Ethiopia. Patients in these countries care more about the location of health facility, hospital comfort and access to appropriate services. Patients perception varies according to education level, age, income and residence.

As indicated by the previous literature, with the increasing population and patient expectation, patient satisfaction analysis is essential to evaluate the accessibility and quality of medical service, especially in developing countries such as China. Some researchers have explored the outpatient satisfaction and factors influencing Chinese patients' satisfaction, mostly from developed provinces or tertiary hospitals. Questionnaire is a commonly used satisfaction survey instrument. As reported in studies conducting univariate or regression analysis, factors including hospital environment, medical facility, service attitude, patients' involvement in decision making, doctors' and nurses' proficient skills, effective communication between patients and doctors, disease severity, medical cost, waiting time and service time are associated with Chinese outpatients' satisfaction in advanced areas or tertiary hospitals.

Chapter 3   Methodology

3.1   Research objectives

Patient perception of health care service presented the effectiveness, safety and benefit of healthcare service, and it can be concluded from the patient decision process, which mainly include the choice of health care provider and satisfaction after medical service. Therefore, patient choice of care providers and satisfaction analysis are important indicators in measuring healthcare service performance, promoting patient satisfaction and improving efficient resource allocation.

Most of China's existing analysis of patient perception were conducted in developed areas and tertiary hospitals, and no questionnaire study had been performed to assess outpatient's satisfaction and choice of care providers with a large-sample evidence covering different backward provinces in China. Considering the relatively lower education level, less individual income and heavier economic burden, it is necessary to process a region-specific questionnaire survey for the outpatient's evaluation and perception of health care service performance in rural western China. Consequently, the specific objectives of this study include:

(1) To investigate the outpatient choice of health care providers for common illness in rural western China;

(2) To analyze the internal factors that influence outpatients' choice of care providers;

(3) To explore the external factors that influence outpatients' choice of

care providers;

(4) To assess the outpatient satisfaction and its dimensionality in rural western China;

(5) To study the factors that influence outpatients' satisfaction in rural western China.

3.2　Research design

3.2.1　Outpatient choice of health care providers in rural western China

To achieve the specific Objective (1), a questionnaire was designed, which included outpatient choice of care providers of common diseases and the internal and external reasons associated with the choice. Outpatient choice was explored through a single-choice question. Participant characteristics were investigated as internal factors, including demographic information, medical insurance types and chronic disease conditions. External factors were analyzed through a multiple-choice question. The outpatient choice of care providers would be calculated based on the survey data.

For the specific Objective (2), further analysis was conducted using the results of the specific Objective (1) and outpatient characteristics. A multinomial logistic regression was performed to assess the association between the internal reasons and outpatient choice of care providers.

To achieve the specific Objective (3), the external reasons that influence outpatient health-seeking choice were investigated using the results of the specific Objective (1) and the answers of multiple-choice question. The multiple response analysis was conducted through SPSS to assess the frequencies of main external reasons associated with outpatient choice of care provider. And the Chi-square test was conducted to investigate the association between external reasons and outpatients' health-seeking choice.

The first questionnaire draft was developed based on the literature review. CNKI and PubMed database were searched in June 2014, using keywords include "outpatient" "choice" "health seeking behavior" "health care demand" "China" and "questionnaire". About 30 previous outpatients' choice analysis and relevant studies were screened. According to existing studies, internal reasons such as occupation, income, education level, medical insurance coverage, marriage status, residence and illness severity were associated with patients' choice of care providers, and external factors including the hospital distance, service attitude, doctors' and nurses' professional skills, drug availability and medical cost were considered associated with Chinese outpatient choice of care providers in urban areas and tertiary hospitals.

To predict the acceptability and feasibility of the questionnaire, and to improve the design quality and efficiency, the pilot study was conducted with a small-size population. Local reimbursement percentage, medical price, residents' income, education level and clinical opinions were also considered, and corresponding justifications were made after the pilot study.

In the final draft version (see Appendix I), health care provider choice was designed as a single-choice question, which contained three options, including the village clinics, the township health centers, and the county and higher-level hospitals. Interviewees were asked to fill their background information including the gender, age, education level, occupation, monthly income, medical insurance type and condition of chronic diseases, which were also investigated as internal factors influencing outpatients' health seeking behavior. External factors were analyzed through a multiple-choice question, with 10 options including "Hospital distance" "Rational medical charges" "Doctors' and nurses' professional skills" "Hospital facility" "Drug supply" "Hospital staff service attitude" "Medical insurance covered hospital" "Knowing somebody work in hospital" "Trustworthy doctor", and "Other reasons".

See details of the development process of outpatient choice questionnaire in Figure 3-1.

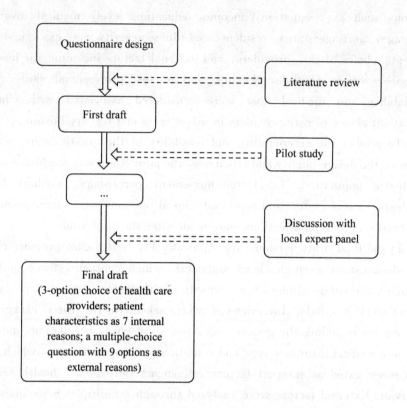

Figure 3-1 Outpatient choice questionnaire development

3.2.2 Outpatient satisfaction in rural western China

To achieve the specific Objective (4), the questionnaire concerning outpatient satisfaction was conducted, investigating satisfaction scores of several outpatient service items and interviewee characteristics including demographic information, medical insurance types and chronic disease conditions. Outpatient satisfaction item scores were calculated, and the dimensionality and structure of overall satisfaction were assessed through Exploratory Factor Analysis.

For the specific Objective (5), further analysis was processed using the results of the specific Objective (4) and outpatient characteristics. The association between the overall and dimensional satisfaction was evaluated through univariate and multilinear regression analysis, using outpatient characteristics as independent variables, and factors scores of dimensional and overall satisfaction as dependent variables.

Literature were reviewed before the design of first draft, literature search was conducted with the CNKI and PubMed database in June 2014, with keywords "outpatient" "satisfaction" "China" and "questionnaire". More than 50 previous outpatients' satisfaction survey and relevant studies were reviewed, the adaptive information was extracted to compose the item pool. As reported in existing studies in advanced areas or tertiary hospitals, factors including hospital environment, medical facility, patients' participation in decision making, patient-doctor communication, medical staff service attitude, doctors' and nurses' proficient skills, disease severity, medical cost, waiting time and service time were the main items constitute Chinese outpatients' satisfaction.

After the pilot study, local medical price, reimbursement percentage, residents' income and education level were considered, and the final draft version was developed after the discussion with local expert panel.

The outpatient service satisfaction survey contains 9 items, including time spent in commuting to hospital, outpatients' waiting time, doctors' disease description, patients' participation in decision making, staff service attitude, hospital facility, hospital environment, medical cost, and doctor and nurses' professional skills. The questionnaire was designed as a five-point Likert scale, and interviewees were asked to rate each item: very dissatisfied (1), dissatisfied (2), neither satisfied nor dissatisfied (3), satisfied (4) and very satisfied (5). The results would be calculated to describe the outpatient satisfaction of each item, based on which analysis of the structure and dimensionality of overall satisfaction would be done.

Interviewees were also asked to fill their background information, including age, gender, occupation, education level, monthly income, medical insurance type and condition of chronic diseases, which would be assessed as potential factors associated with dimensional and overall outpatient satisfaction.

The development process of outpatient satisfaction questionnaire is shown in Figure 3-2.

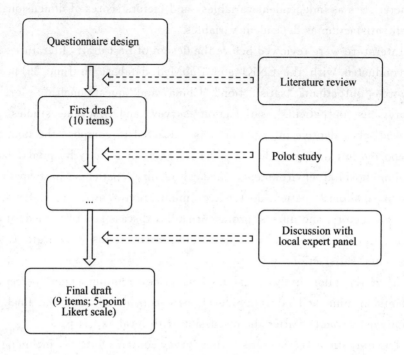

Figure 3-2　Outpatient satisfaction questionnaire development

3.3　Data source

3.3.1　Field study

The field study in rural western China was conducted from October to December, 2014. Eleven provincial-level divisions in western China were chosen as sample provinces, including Ningxia, Guangxi, Xinjiang, Gansu, Shaanxi, Qinghai, Sichuan, Guizhou, Yunnan, Inner Mongolia and Tibet.

western China is a relatively poorer district. At the end of 2014, the population of these 11 western provinces was nearly 338.48 million, accounting for 1/4 of China's total population (1.37 billion), while the GDP of western China represented only 19.2% of the nationally total amount. The GDP per capital of western China in 2014 was only 37,487 *yuan*, less than

66, 960 *yuan* of eastern China and 39,098 *yuan* of middle China.[1]

Healthcare workforce shortage was also observed in backward areas. In 2016, the number of licensed physicians per 10 thousand residents in western China was 21.75, less than the 26.09 in eastern China and the 22.13 in middle China. While the number of registered nurses per 10 thousand residents in western China was only 24, much less than the 28.45 in eastern China.[2]

To investigate the patient perception of health care service in backward areas, outpatients in rural western China were selected to explore the health care service satisfaction and choice of care provider.

3.3.2 Literature and document review

Official reports and data from international organizations including WHO and World Bank were reviewed as reference. To get a better understanding of the health care resource utilization in rural and urban China, statistical yearbooks from National Health Commission of PRC, NHC (formerly known as National Health and Family Planning Commission of PRC, NHFPC), National Bureau of Statistics, and the third and fourth National Health Service Survey reports were also referred to.

3.4 Data collection and sampling

To avoid the selection bias caused by the economic condition, all counties in each province were divided into three levels according to GDP per capita, and one sample county was randomly selected from each level of these 11 provinces. The local county general hospital, the county maternal and child health center (MCH), the county hospital of traditional Chinese medicine (TCM) in each sample county were chosen as sample county hospitals, and 2-3 township health centers in each sample county were systematically selected as sample township hospitals.

Questionnaires were conducted in a total of 160 healthcare institutions, including 30 county general hospitals, 23 county MCHs, 21 county hospitals of TCM and 86 township health centers. Due to the lack of data in some

---

① Data source: National Bureau of Statistics of China.
② Data source: National Bureau of Statistics of China.

regions, the number of sample county hospitals and sample township health centers varied in each province.

See details of the number and distribution of sample hospitals in Table 3-1 below.

Table 3-1   Number and distribution of sample health care institutions

	No. of sample health care institutions				
	Township health center	County general hospital	County MCH	County hospital of TCM	Total
Gansu	9	3	3	2	17
Guangxi	9	3	3	3	18
Guizhou	9	3	0	0	12
Inner Mongolia	5	2	2	2	11
Ningxia	7	3	3	3	16
Qinghai	4	1	1	2	8
Shaanxi	6	3	2	3	14
Sichuan	9	3	3	3	18
Tibet	9	3	0	0	12
Xinjiang	9	3	3	1	16
Yunnan	10	3	3	2	18
Total	86	30	23	21	160

Considering that the average numbers of daily outpatient visits in county-level hospitals were higher than those of township health centers, 50 outpatients from each county hospital and 30 patients from each township health center were enrolled into the questionnaire. Written informed consents (see Appendix II) was obtained from all interviewees before filling the questionnaire.

About 50 investigators were recruited before the survey. After a systematic training, investigators were divided into two groups, being assigned to distribute questionnaires in the outpatient area of every sample healthcare institutions. Outpatients received the questionnaire before leaving the hospital, with all questions explained by trained investigators. The questionnaire for interviewees under 14 were completed by his/her adult supervisor.

3.5   Data process and statistical analysis

3.5.1   Method used to describe patient characteristics and choice of care providers

Descriptive data were calculated to present the distribution of participants and interviewees' characteristics, including:

(1) Number and percentage of outpatient from township health centers, county general hospitals, county MCHs and county hospitals of TCM;

(2) Number and percentage of outpatient with different genders, education levels, occupations, monthly income, medical insurance types and chronic disease conditions;

(3) Interviewees' mean age, number and percentage of outpatients in each age groups.

The Chi-square test was adopted to explore the difference between interviewees from township health centers and county-level hospitals, with $p < 0.05$.

The number and percentage of participants who chose village clinic, the number and percentage of participants who chose the township health center and the number and percentage of participants who chose the county and higher-level hospital were calculated to describe outpatient health-seeking choice based on the survey data.

3.5.2   Method used to assess internal reasons associated with outpatient choice of care providers

In this study, interviewees' characteristics were evaluated as internal reasons. Univariate analysis and multinomial logistic regression analysis were conducted to assess the association between internal reasons and outpatient choice of health care providers.

Univariate logistic regression analysis was performed to investigate the statistical significance between outpatients' each internal reason and their choice of care provider, respectively. Then participant characteristics which showed significant differences in the univariate analysis were included in the multinomial logistic regression model as independent variables, and outpatients' choices as dependent variables. The odds ratios (OR) was adopted to indicate the negative or positive association between internal reasons and the outpatient health-seeking choice, and the p values were used to quantify the statistical significance, which was deemed to be at a 95% confidence level (CI) or $p < 0.05$.

3.5.3 Method used to assess external reasons associated with outpatient choice of care providers

The multiple response analysis and Chi-square test were processed to investigate the association between external reasons and outpatients' choice of health care provider in rural western China.

The multiple response analysis by SPSS was adopted to interpret the result of the multiple-choice question, showing the frequencies and percentage of interviewees who made choice. The most frequently chosen external reasons would be considered as the primary external reasons that influence outpatient the choice of care provider in rural western China.

A comparison of outpatient who made different choices on each option was made through Chi-square test, to investigate the association between main external factors and outpatient characteristics. The between-group statistical significance was set at a 95% confidence interval (CI) or $p < 0.05$. The adjusted residuals (AR) that exceeds about 3 in Chi-square tests were used to interpret the in-group difference of each cell.

3.5.4 Method used to assess outpatient satisfaction item scores

The mean scores and standard deviation (SD) was calculated to present outpatient satisfaction of each item.

3.5.5 Method used to assess the dimensionality of outpatient satisfaction

Exploratory factor analysis was performed to explore the dimensionality of the overall outpatients' satisfaction, analyze the validity of the dimensional structure, and reduce the number of variables.

Before the factor analysis, the Cronbach's alpha coefficient was tested to evaluate the overall reliability of the data set, which was considered acceptable with the value more than 0.7. The Bartlett's test of sphericity, the Kaiser-Meyer-Olkin (KMO) value and the Measure of Sample Adequacy (MSA) of the Anti-Image Correlation Matrices was used to measure the sampling adequacy for factor analysis. The data set would be considered appropriate for EFA with the KMO value more than 0.6 and the significant result of Bartlett's test of sphericity, while values in the Anti-Image Matrices should be above 0.5.

The principal component analysis was done to extract the factors and calculate the unrotated factor loadings, which determined the dimensional structure of the data set. The variable (outpatient satisfaction item) with initial community less than 0.2 would be deleted from the data set. According to Pallant (2013), the EFA dimensional structure should adopt a solution not only with as few factors as possible, but also can explain the variance as much as possible. The number of factors with eigenvalues greater than 1 (the Kaiser's criterion), the number of factors before the horizontal curve in the scree plot and parallel analysis were commonly used approaches to determine the number of factors. While the percentage of cumulative variance and the number of non-trivial factors were also commonly used indicators. In this study, the Kaiser's criterion, the scree test results and the percentage of cumulative variance were considered to determine the number of factors.

In this study, the varimax rotation with Kaisa Normalization was adopted as the rotative solution to interpret the extracted factors. Rotated factor loadings in the component matrix could tell the relative contribution of each item to factors, and the rotation solution would be tested by the Component Correlation Matrix, which demonstrated the strength of the relationship between each factor.

The reliability and internal consistency of each extracted factor were evaluated by using Cronbach's alpha coefficient and inter-item correlation. The factor consistency would be rated good reliability with the Cronbach's alpha value more than 0.7. When the number of items in the scale was less than 10, Cronbach's alpha value would be quite small, and the inter item correlation (IIC) for the items should be reported as the primary measure of internal consistency, with the acceptable mean IIC value ranging from 0.2 to 0.4.

3.5.6 Method used to assess the factors that influence dimensional and overall outpatient satisfaction

The univariate analysis was conducted to evaluate the association between outpatient characteristics and outpatient satisfaction factor scores, including ANOVA analysis, t-test, Spearman correlation test and Pearson correlation test. The stepwise multi-linear regressive analysis was performed to explore the influencing factors of dimensional and overall outpatient satisfaction, using the overall satisfaction factor score and dimensional factor score as dependent variables. However, outpatient characteristics showed significant differences in the univariate analysis were included as independent variables.

In this study, the regression method was adopted to estimate the factor score coefficients, which represented the relationship between variables and factors. And the factor scores were calculated by using factor score coefficients with weights in equation below (F_i: the score of $Factor_i$; β_{ni}: factor score coefficients of $Factor_i$; $Variable_{ni}$: score of items constitute $Factor_i$; ϵ_i: residual):

$$F_i = \beta_{1i} * Variable_{1i} + \beta_{2i} * Variable_{2i} + \cdots + \beta_{ni} * Variable_{ni} + \epsilon_i$$

The factor score of overall satisfaction was calculated based on the dimensional factor score and the variance contribution rate (F: the factor scores of overall satisfactions; $Variance_i$: the variance explained by $Factor_i$):

$$F = Variance_1 * F_1 + Variance_2 * F_2 + \cdots + Variance_i * F_i$$

After the weight calculation, the overall satisfaction score of each participant could also be calculated based on the overall satisfaction factor score equation and cumulative variance rate. (Field, 2013)

Chapter 4   Result I : Outpatients' choices of care providers in rural western China

The questionnaire survey was conducted from October to December, 2014. A total of 4,616 outpatients participated in the survey, and 4,233 questionnaires were fully completed. The total response rate was 91.7%.

Table 4-1 shows the geographical distribution of participants.

Table 4-1   **The distribution of participants**

	Hospital type				Total
	Township health center	County general hospital	County MCH	County hospital of TCM	
Gansu	241	119	78	76	514
Guangxi	224	116	145	125	610
Guizhou	94	76	0	0	170
Inner Mongolia	54	91	47	62	254
Ningxia	98	101	36	71	306
Qinghai	96	3	41	63	203
Shaanxi	53	110	33	85	281
Sichuan	261	108	101	127	597
Tibet	230	152	0	0	382
Xinjiang	217	93	72	39	421
Yunnan	228	126	91	50	495
Total	1,796	1,095	644	698	4,233

1,796 respondents (42.4%) came from 86 township health centers; 1,095 respondents (25.7%) came from 30 county general hospitals; 644 outpatients (15.2%) came from 23 county maternal and child health centers (MCH); and 698 outpatients (16.5%) came from 21 county hospital of traditional Chinese medicine (TCM). Due to the lack of data in some autonomous areas of ethnic minorities in Guizhou, Qinghai and Tibet, the sample size varied in each province, and the geographic differences were taken into consideration in the exploration of internal factors.

4.1 Descriptive findings

The result of outpatients' choice of health care providers shows that 1,928 participants (45.5%) would visit township health centers to cure common illness, 747 responders (17.6%) chose village clinics as the preferred health care provider, and 1,558 interviewees (36.8%) selected county and higher-level hospital as the first option.

The descriptive results of participants' demographic and other background characteristics are demonstrated in Table 4-2. Of all 4,233 respondents, 56.8% were female, and 67% of participants' ages ranged from 25 to 54. Only 30% of interviewees had completed high school education or got more higher degrees. Farmer was the most common occupation, and 73.1% of respondents' income was less than 2,001 *yuan* (about $330) per month. Most participants were enrolled in public medical insurance system; 11.6% of respondents were insured by Urban Employee Basic Medical Insurance; 6.6% were insured by Urban Resident Basic Medical Insurance; and 70.9% insured by New Rural Cooperative Medical Scheme. 25% of the participants had chronic diseases.

Table 4-2 **Respondents' characteristics**

Characteristics			No.	%
Gender	Female		2,404	56.8
	Male		1,829	43.2
Age	≤14		73	1.7
	15-24		551	13.0
	25-34		1,225	28.9

Continued

Characteristics		No.	%
Age	35-44	890	21.0
	45-54	725	17.1
	55-64	439	10.4
	≥65	330	7.8
Education	Illiteracy	601	14.2
	Primary school	981	23.2
	Junior high school	1,381	32.6
	High school	775	18.3
	College or above	495	11.7
Occupation	Farmer	1,963	46.4
	Blue-collar worker	463	10.9
	Business/Service	585	13.8
	Teacher/Government staff	382	9.0
	Student/Unemployment/Other jobs	756	17.9
	Retirement	84	2.0
Monthly income	No income	1,112	26.3
	1-2,000 *yuan*	1,980	46.8
	2,001-4,000 *yuan*	901	21.3
	4,001 *yuan* and above	240	5.7
Medical insurance	National health insurance	114	2.7
	UEBMI	491	11.6
	URBMI	278	6.6
	NRCMS	3,000	70.9
	Medical insurance for urban and rural residents①	93	2.2
	Other insurances	55	1.3
	No insurance	202	4.8

① This insurance scheme was launched at the beginning of 1992 mainly in the western provinces in China. It's different from the Basic Medical Insurance for Urban and Rural Residents launched in April. 2009, which include UEBMI, URBMI and NRCMS. For some special reasons, this insurance scheme is still used by some residents in the rural western area in China.

Continued

Characteristics		No.	%
Chronic diseases	Yes	1,046	24.7
	No	3,187	75.3

Table 4-3 shows the descriptive findings of different sample hospital levels. According to the Chi-square tests, statistical significances were observed between township health centers and county-level hospitals in the distribution of education level, occupation, monthly income, medical insurance type, and chronic disease conditions, with all p values less than 0.001. The proportion of female outpatients (60.0%) in county-level hospitals was higher than township health centers (52.4%, $p < 0.001$). Interviewees from township health centers were elder than these from county-level hospitals, because 62.3% of interviewees from county-level hospitals were older than 35 years old. Only 18.9% of respondents from township health centers accepted high school education or got higher degrees, and high school achievement rate of outpatients from county-level hospitals was 38.2%. 60% of participants from township health centers were farmers, while the proportion of farmers from county-level hospitals was 36.8%. 23% of outpatient from township health centers and 30% from county-level hospitals earned more than 2,001 *yuan* (about \$330) per month, respectively. About 82% of respondents from township health centers were insured by New Rural Cooperative Medical Scheme, higher than the 62.8% of county-level hospitals. The chronic disease prevalence of participants from township health centers was 30.1%, which is higher than the 20.1% of county-level hospitals.

Table 4-3　Respondents' characteristics according to sample hospital levels

Characteristics	Township health centers N=1,796	County-level hospitals N=2,437
Gender ($p < 0.001$)		
Female	941(52.4%)	1,463(60.0%)
Male	855(47.6%)	974(40.0%)

Continued

Characteristics	Township health centers N=1,796	County-level hospitals N=2,437
Age　(*p*<0.001)		
≤14	33(1.8%)	40(1.6%)
15-24	185(10.3%)	366(15.0%)
25-34	425(23.7%)	800(32.8%)
35-44	383(21.3%)	507(20.8%)
45-54	339(18.9%)	386(15.8%)
55-64	233(13.0%)	206(8.5%)
≥65	198(11.0%)	132(5.4%)
Education　(*p*<0.001)		
Illiteracy	343(19.1%)	258(10.6%)
Primary school	499(27.8%)	482(19.8%)
Junior high school	615(34.2%)	766(31.4%)
High school	229(12.8%)	546(22.4%)
College and above	110(6.1%)	385(15.8%)
Occupation　(*p*<0.001)		
Farmer	1,066(59.4%)	896(36.8%)
Blue-collar worker	193(10.7%)	270(11.1%)
Business/Service	175(9.7%)	410(16.8%)
Teacher/Government staff	108(6.0%)	274(11.2%)
Student/Unemployment/ Other jobs	222(12.4%)	534(21.9%)
Retirement	32(1.8%)	52(2.1%)
Monthly income　(*p*<0.001)		
No income	533(29.7%)	579(23.8%)
1-2,000 *yuan*	856(47.7%)	1,124(46.1%)
2,001-4,000 *yuan*	315(17.5%)	586(24.0%)
4,001 *yuan* and more	92(5.1%)	148(6.1%)

Continued

Characteristics	Township health centers N=1,796	County-level hospitals N=2,437
Medical insurance （$p<0.001$）		
National health insurance	30(1.7%)	84(3.4%)
UEBMI	122(6.8%)	369(15.1%)
URBMI	75(4.2%)	203(8.3%)
NRCMS	1,469(81.8%)	1,531(62.8%)
Medical insurance for urban and rural residents	34(1.9%)	59(2.4%)
Other insurances	18(1.0%)	37(1.5%)
No insurance	48(2.7%)	154(6.3%)
Chronic diseases （$p<0.001$）		
Yes	556(31.0%)	490(20.1%)
No	1,240(69.0%)	1,947(79.9%)

4.2　Internal factors associated with outpatients' choices

Nine internal characteristics, including the sample hospital type, province, age, gender, education, occupation, monthly income, the type of medical insurance and the condition of chronic diseases, show significant differences in the univariate logistic regression respectively. See details in Table 4-4.

Table 4-4　　　　　　Univariate logistic regression

Variables	-2 Log Likelyhood	DF	p
Hospital type	54.348	6	<0.001
Age	86.828	12	<0.001

Continued

Variables	-2 Log Likelyhood	DF	p
Gender	30.380	2	<0.001
Medical insurance	73.999	12	<0.001
Occupation	70.719	10	<0.001
Province	129.357	20	<0.001
Monthly income	53.011	6	<0.001
Education	65.037	8	<0.001
Chronic diseases	30.380	2	<0.001

The multinomial logistic regression results are presented in Table 4-5. The odds ratios and p values indicate that 7 internal factors including sample hospital type, province, gender, education, occupation, monthly income and health insurance type were significantly associated with outpatients' choice of health care providers in rural western China.

Compared with county hospitals of TCM, outpatients from township health centers would like to visit township health centers first, then village clinics, but outpatients from county MCHs preferred higher-level hospitals rather than village clinics.

In Gansu, Inner Mongolia, Qinghai, Shaanxi and Xinjiang, outpatients chose to visit village clinics to cure common diseases, and outpatients from Guangxi prefer county and higher-level hospitals.

Male patients tend to consider village or township health centers as the primary option.

Compared with respondents who have completed college or higher education, the primary options of outpatients with lower education to cure common diseases was village clinics, and then they chose township health centers; county and higher-level hospitals were the last choice.

Outpatients with different occupations also chose different health care providers. Village clinics were the primary option of farmers and blue-collar workers; teachers and government staffs preferred township health centers to village clinics; students, the unemployed and outpatients with other jobs preferred village clinics to township health centers.

To outpatients who earned less than 4,000 *yuan* per month, the first choice to cure common diseases was village clinics, then township health centers; county and higher-level hospitals were the last choice. The less the monthly incomes, the more significant the differences.

Taking respondents with no medical insurance as reference category, outpatients with Urban Employee Basic Medical Insurance preferred county and higher-level hospitals, while outpatients with Urban Resident Basic Medical Insurance preferred county and higher-level hospitals to village clinics, and outpatients insured by New Rural Cooperative Medical Scheme preferred township health centers to village clinics.

Table 4-5

Multinomial logistic regression results

	Village clinics vs. County and higher-level hospitals			County and higher-level hospitals vs. Township health centers			Township health centers vs. Village clinics		
	OR	95% CI	p	OR	95% CI	p	OR	95% CI	p
Hospital type (County hospital of TCM as reference category)									
Township health center	4.795	3.478-6.609	<0.001***	0.114	0.088-0.148	<0.001***	1.825	1.387-2.403	<0.001***
County general hospital	0.934	0.675-1.293	0.682	1.213	0.941-1.562	0.136	0.882	0.644-1.210	0.438
County MCH	0.648	0.439-0.955	0.028*	0.897	0.682-1.179	0.435	1.722	1.183-2.507	0.005**
Province (Yunnan Province as reference category)									
Gansu	4.234	2.724-6.582	<0.001***	0.614	0.428-0.881	0.008**	0.385	0.269-0.550	<0.001***
Guangxi	0.481	0.305-0.759	0.002**	1.850	1.347-2.540	<0.001***	1.123	0.742-1.700	0.583
Guizhou	0.872	0.453-1.678	0.682	0.853	0.524-1.389	0.523	1.344	0.770-2.344	0.298
Inner Mongolia	3.517	2.094-5.906	<0.001***	0.551	0.360-0.843	0.006**	0.516	0.335-0.796	0.003**
Ningxia	1.217	0.716-2.017	0.468	1.408	0.938-2.113	0.099	0.584	0.360-0.946	0.029*
Qinghai	8.592	4.658-15.849	<0.001***	0.534	0.303-0.941	0.030*	0.218	0.143-0.333	<0.001***
Shaanxi	2.035	1.249-3.314	0.004**	1.027	0.691-1.528	0.894	0.478	0.309-0.742	0.001**
Sichuan	1.155	0.728-1.833	0.540	0.837	0.597-1.172	0.300	1.034	0.694-1.541	0.868
Tibet	0.515	0.310-0.853	0.010**	1.443	0.990-2.106	0.057	1.346	0.871-2.080	0.180

Continued

	Village clinics vs. County and higher-level hospitals			County and higher-level hospitals vs. Township health centers			Township health centers vs. Village clinics		
	OR	95% CI	p	OR	95% CI	p	OR	95% CI	p
Xinjiang	1.965	1.218-3.170	0.006**	1.061	0.738-1.524	0.750	0.480	0.317-0.727	0.001**
Gender (Female as reference category)									
Male	1.368	1.096-1.708	0.006**	0.759	0.637-0.905	0.002**	0.963	0.798-1.161	0.691
Age ($\geq$65 as reference category)									
$\leqslant$14	0.630	0.274-1.449	0.277	1.772	0.838-3.747	0.134	0.896	0.437-1.838	0.764
15-24	0.729	0.408-1.301	0.284	1.058	0.656-1.706	0.817	1.297	0.806-2.089	0.284
25-34	0.815	0.488-1.361	0.435	1.004	0.646-1.563	0.985	1.221	0.823-1.811	0.321
35-44	0.884	0.536-1.459	0.630	1.161	0.747-1.804	0.506	0.974	0.668-1.419	0.890
45-54	0.897	0.544-1.480	0.670	1.078	0.690-1.684	0.742	1.034	0.716-1.494	0.857
55-64	0.699	0.414-1.179	0.179	1.278	0.806-2.028	0.297	1.120	0.764-1.642	0.562
Education (College and above as reference category)									
Illiteracy	9.208	4.607-18.404	<0.001***	0.346	0.222-0.539	<0.001***	0.314	0.162-0.607	0.001**
Primary school	5.262	2.713-10.206	<0.001***	0.430	0.292-0.634	<0.001***	0.442	0.231-0.843	0.013*
Junior high school	2.840	1.516-5.322	0.001**	0.662	0.472-0.930	0.017*	0.532	0.284-0.996	0.049*

Continued

	Village clinics vs. County and higher-level hospitals			County and higher-level hospitals vs. Township health centers			Township health centers vs. Village clinics		
	OR	95% CI	p	OR	95% CI	p	OR	95% CI	p
High school	2.069	1.097-3.901	0.025*	0.756	0.545-1.048	0.093	0.639	0.337-1.213	0.171
Occupation (Retirement as reference category)									
Farmer	11.435	2.489-52.541	0.002**	0.476	0.252-0.898	0.022*	0.184	0.041-0.820	0.026*
Blue-collar worker	10.466	2.229-49.136	0.003**	0.540	0.279-1.046	0.068	0.177	0.039-0.804	0.025*
Business/Service/Enterprise employee	3.549	0.748-16.846	0.111	1.085	0.567-2.075	0.806	0.260	0.056-1.201	0.085
Teacher/Government staff	4.740	0.927-24.229	0.062	1.070	0.544-2.105	0.844	0.197	0.039-0.991	0.049*
Student/Unemployment/Others	5.538	1.172-26.158	0.031*	0.817	0.421-1.585	0.550	0.221	0.048-1.016	0.052
Monthly income (4,001 yuan and above as reference category)									
No income	5.644	2.985-10.672	<0.001***	0.429	0.282-0.653	<0.001***	0.413	0.224-0.761	0.005**
1-2,000 yuan	3.441	1.879-6.305	<0.001***	0.366	0.252-0.532	<0.001***	0.794	0.439-1.438	0.447
2,001-4,000 yuan	1.559	0.822-2.957	0.174	0.529	0.361-0.774	0.001**	1.214	0.646-2.281	0.547
Medical insurance (No insurance as reference category)									
National health insurance	0.528	0.218-1.278	0.157	1.631	0.862-3.086	0.133	1.160	0.478-2.819	0.743

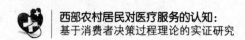

Continued

	Village clinics vs. County and higher-level hospitals			County and higher-level hospitals vs. Township health centers			Township health centers vs. Village clinics		
	OR	95% CI	p	OR	95% CI	p	OR	95% CI	p
UEBMI	0.228	0.113-0.462	<0.001***	1.788	1.123-2.846	0.014*	2.450	1.220-4.919	0.012*
URBMI	0.166	0.077-0.355	<0.001***	1.570	0.976-2.527	0.063	3.847	1.811-8.173	<0.001***
NRCMS	0.855	0.541-1.352	0.503	0.722	0.495-1.053	0.091	1.619	1.040-2.521	0.033*
Medical insurance for urban and rural residents	0.809	0.356-1.838	0.613	1.045	0.554-1.971	0.892	1.183	0.543-2.579	0.673
Other insurances	0.403	0.128-1.267	0.120	1.226	0.574-2.621	0.598	2.023	0.650-6.295	0.224
Chronic diseases (Yes as reference category)									
No	1.111	0.855-1.444	0.432	0.863	0.698-1.068	0.176	1.043	0.839-1.296	0.707

* $p<0.05$, ** $p<0.01$, *** $p<0.001$

4.3 External factors associated with outpatients' choices

A multiple-choice question was answered by 4,233 participants to investigate the external reasons that influence outpatients' health seeking behavior, and an average of 1.87 options were chosen by each outpatient. The results of SPSS multiple response analysis indicate that "hospital distance" (33.2%), "rational medical charge"(16.3%), "hospital staff service attitude" (11.8%) and doctors' and nurses' professional skills" (11.6%) were the main four external factors that influence the choice of primary health care outpatients from rural western China, which were considered by 61.9%, 30.4%, 22.0% and 12.6% of participants as the primary external reason respectively.

The main external reasons are presented in Figure 4-1.

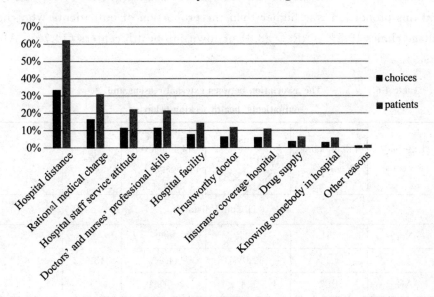

Figure 4-1 The external reasons

Table 4-6 shows the association between external reasons and outpatients' health seeking behavior, and the p values and ARs (adjusted residual) of Chi-square tests present that outpatients' choices of health care provider were significantly associated with the main four external reasons. With all p values lower than 0.001, and some ARs exceeding about 3, significant differences of external reasons were observed among outpatients who selected different care providers.

Most respondents who chose village clinics (79.1%, AR = 10.7) and township health centers (69.6%, AR = 9.4) cared about "hospital distance", and their proportion was significantly higher than that of respondents who chose county and higher-level hospitals (44.2%, AR = −18.1). More participants who chose township health centers believed that "rational medical charge" was a crucial factor (37.4%, AR = 9.0). Only 13.9% of outpatients considered about "hospital staff service attitude" when they visited village clinics (AR = −5.9), and this proportion was significantly lower than that of outpatients who chose county and higher-level hospital (24.5%, AR = 2.9). Around 1/3 of outpatients who tended to visit county and higher-level hospitals believed that "doctors' and nurses' professional skills" was the most dominant factor when they sought health care services (35.9%, AR = 17.2), and this proportion was higher than the proportion of outpatients who chose village clinics (9.5%, AR = −8.8) or township health centers (14.7%, AR = −9.9).

Table 4-6　　　The association between external reasons and
outpatients' health seeking behavior

External Reasons	Village clinic (N=747)	Township health center (N=1,928)	County and higher-level hospital (N=1,558)	χ^2	p
Hospital distance					
No.	591	1,342	689	348.992	<0.001***
%	79.1%	69.6%	44.2%		
AR	10.7	9.4	−18.1		
Rational medical charge					
No.	195	721	371	83.064	<0.001***
%	26.1%	37.4%	23.8%		
AR	−2.8	9.0	−7.1		

Continued

External Reasons	Village clinic (N=747)	Township health center (N=1,928)	County and higher-level hospital (N=1,558)	χ^2	p
Hospital staff service attitude					
No.	104	447	381	35.429	<0.001***
%	13.9%	23.2%	24.5%		
AR	−5.9	1.7	2.9		
Doctors' and nurses' professional skills					
No.	71	284	559	305.934	<0.001***
%	9.5%	14.7%	35.9%		
AR	−8.8	−9.9	17.2		

The association between patient characteristics and external factors were evaluated by univariate analysis. The Chi-square test results present that respondents' gender, age, income, education level, occupation, medical insurance type and chronic disease conditions were also significantly associated with at least one dominant external reasons.

More male patients (63.8%) considered "hospital distance" as the dominant external factor than females (60.6%, p=0.035). See details in Table 4-7.

Table 4-7   Main external reasons in different genders

	Male (N=1,829)	Female (N=2,404)	χ^2	p
Hospital distance				
No.	1,166	1,456	4.47	0.035
%	63.80%	60.60%		
AR	2.1	−2.1		

Continued

	Male (N=1,829)	Female (N=2,404)	χ^2	p
Rational medical charge				
No.	576	711		
%	31.50%	29.60%	1.804	0.179
AR	1.3	−1.3		
Hospital staff service attitude				
No.	408	524		
%	22.30%	21.80%	0.158	0.691
AR	0.4	−0.4		
Doctors' and nurses' professional skills				
No.	384	530		
%	21.00%	22.00%	0.678	0.41
AR	−0.8	0.8		

Main external reasons in different occupations are presented in Table 4-8. Farmers (69.10%, AR = 9.0) cared more about hospital distance than teachers/government staff (52.6%, AR = − 3.9) and service industry/ business industry/enterprise employees (48.0%, AR = − 7.5), while the farmers cared less about "doctors' and nurses' professional skills" (15.6%, AR=−8.8) than teachers/governments staffs (29.8%, AR=4.1) and service industry/business industry/enterprise employees (28.9%, AR=4.6).

Table 4-8   **Main external reasons in different occupations**

		Farmer (N=1,963)	Worker (N=463)	Business/Service/ Enterprise employee (N=585)	Teacher/Government staff (N=382)	Student/ Unemployment/ Others (N=756)	Retirement (N=84)	χ^2	p
Hospital distance	No.	1,357	275	281	201	463	45	109.025	<0.001****
	%	69.10%	59.40%	48.00%	52.60%	61.20%	53.60%		
	AR	9	-1.2	-7.5	-3.9	-0.4	-1.6		
Rational medical charge	No.	640	153	181	135	155	23	45.881	<0.001****
	%	32.60%	33.00%	30.90%	35.30%	20.50%	27.40%		
	AR	2.9	1.3	0.3	2.2	-6.5	-0.6		
Hospital staff service attitude	No.	439	100	128	108	135	22	17.368	0.004**
	%	22.40%	21.60%	21.90%	28.30%	17.90%	26.20%		
	AR	0.5	-0.2	-0.1	3.1	-3	0.9		
Doctors' and nurses' professional skills	No.	307	108	169	114	190	26	85.611	<0.001****
	%	15.60%	23.30%	28.90%	29.80%	25.10%	31.00%		
	AR	-8.8	1	4.6	4.1	2.6	2.1		

* $p<0.05$, ** $p<0.01$, **** $p<0.001$.

As shown in Table 4-9, it is significant that more outpatients with chronic diseases considered "rational medical charge" (34.4%, AR=3.3) and "hospital staff service attitude" (26.4%, AR=3.9) than those without chronic diseases. It seems that patients with long-term experience of health problems suffered from heavier disease burden, and was in higher demand of better service attitude than other patients.

Table 4-9   Main external reasons in different chronic disease conditions

External reasons	Without chronic disease (N=3,187)	With chronic disease (N=1,046)	χ^2	p
Hospital distance				
No.	1,962	660		
%	61.60%	63.10%	0.787	0.375
AR	−0.9	0.9		
Rational medical charge				
No.	927	360		
%	29.10%	34.40%	10.573	0.001**
AR	−3.3	3.3		
Hospital staff service attitude				
No.	656	276		
%	20.60%	26.40%	15.444	<0.001***
AR	−3.9	3.9		
Doctors' and nurses' professional skills				
No.	700	214		
%	22.00%	20.50%	1.054	0.305
AR	1.0	−1.0		

* $p<0.05$, ** $p<0.01$, *** $p<0.001$.

According to Table 4-10, more NRCMS-insured respondents (66.2%, AR=8.9) considered "hospital distance" as the most important external reasons than the UEBMI-insured (49.5%, AR=−6.0) and URBMI (51.4%, AR=−3.7), while more public health services insured (36.8%. AR=6.0) and UEBMI-insured (30.8%, AR=5.2) outpatients select "doctors' and nurses' professional skills" than the NRCMS-insured (19.0%, AR=−6.5).

Table 4-10   **Main external reasons in different insurance types**

		National health insurance (N=114)	UEBMI (N=491)	URBMI (N=278)	NRCMS (N=3,000)	Medical insurance for urban and rural residents (N=93)	Other insurances (N=55)	No insurance (N=202)	χ^2	p
Hospital distance	n	63	243	143	1,986	49	25	113	83.336	<0.001***
	%	55.3%	49.5%	51.4%	66.2%	52.7%	45.5%	55.9%		
	AR	-1.5	-6.0	-3.7	8.9	-1.9	-2.5	-1.8		
Rational medical charge	n	46	158	78	912	29	11	53	11.282	0.080
	%	40.4%	32.2%	28.1%	30.4%	31.2%	20.0%	26.2%		
	AR	2.3	0.9	-0.9	0.0	0.2	-1.7	-1.3		
Hospital staff service attitude	n	30	128	60	646	22	9	37	9.142	0.166
	%	26.3%	26.1%	21.6%	21.5%	23.7%	16.4%	18.3%		
	AR	1.1	2.3	-0.2	-1.2	0.4	-1.0	-1.3		
Doctors' and nurses' professional skills	n	42	151	72	569	25	14	41	57.484	<0.001***
	%	36.8%	30.8%	25.9%	19.0%	26.9%	25.5%	20.3%		
	AR	4.0	5.2	1.8	-6.5	1.3	0.7	-0.5		

* $p<0.05$, ** $p<0.01$, *** $p<0.001$.

The Mantel-Haenszel Chi-Square test was performed to assess the relationship between ordinal variables and external factors.

As indicated in Table 4-11, respondents at the age of 45 or older cared more about "hospital distance" ($p < 0.001$), patients younger than 25 cared less about "rational medical charge" ($p = 0.019$), patient older than 45 cared less about the "doctors' and nurses' professional skills" ($p < 0.001$).

Table 4-11　　　　The association between external reasons and outpatients' age

	≤14 (N=73)	15-24 (N=551)	25-34 (N=1,225)	35-44 (N=890)	45-54 (N=725)	55-64 (N=439)	≥65 (N=330)	χ^2	p
Hospital distance									
No.	44	310	691	556	499	301	221	49.936	<0.001***
%	60.30%	56.30%	56.40%	62.50%	68.80%	68.60%	67.00%		
AR	-0.3	-2.9	-4.7	0.4	4.2	3.0	2.0		
Rational medical charge									
No.	12	148	377	280	218	145	107	12.654	0.019*
%	16.40%	26.90%	30.80%	31.50%	30.10%	33.00%	32.40%		
AR	-2.6	-1.9	0.3	0.8	-0.2	1.3	0.8		
Hospital staff service attitude									
No.	14	114	281	187	166	97	73	2.369	0.663
%	19.20%	20.70%	22.90%	21.00%	22.90%	22.10%	22.10%		
AR	-0.6	-0.8	0.9	-0.8	0.6	0.0	0.0		
Doctors' and nurses' professional skills									
No.	19	143	271	211	125	82	63	21.12	<0.001***
%	26.00%	26.00%	22.10%	23.70%	17.20%	18.70%	19.10%		
AR	0.9	2.7	0.5	1.7	-3.1	-1.6	-1.2		

* $p<0.05$, *** $p<0.01$, *** $p<0.001$.

Table 4-12 presents the main external reasons for different income levels. More high-income outpatients considered "doctors' and nurses' professional skills" as crucial external reasons ($p < 0.001$), while more respondants with lower income or no income tended to consider "hospital distance" as one of the most dominant external reasons that determine the choice of care providers ($p < 0.001$).

Table 4-12   **Main external reasons in different monthly income levels**

		Without income (N=1,112)	1-2,000 yuan (N=1,980)	2,001-4,000 yuan (N=901)	≥4,001 yuan (N=240)	χ^2	p
Hospital distance	No.	741	1,255	519	107	50.016	<0.001***
	%	66.60%	63.40%	57.60%	44.60%		
	AR	3.8	1.8	-3	-5.7		
Rational medical charge	No.	332	580	294	81	4.693	0.091
	%	29.90%	29.30%	32.60%	33.80%		
	AR	-0.5	-1.5	1.6	1.2		
Hospital staff service attitude	No.	257	419	200	56	1.879	0.851
	%	23.10%	21.20%	22.20%	23.30%		
	AR	1	-1.3	0.1	0.5		
Doctors' and nurses' professional skills	No.	215	383	228	88	48.813	<0.001***
	%	19.30%	19.30%	25.30%	36.70%		
	AR	-2.1	-3.3	3.1	5.8		

* $p<0.05$, ** $p<0.01$, *** $p<0.001$.

The comparison of main internal reasons among different education levels is shown in Table 4-13. More outpatients with higher level of education cared about "hospital staff attitude" ($p < 0.001$) and "doctors' and nurses' professional skills" ($p < 0.001$), while respondants with lower education cared more about "hospital distance" ($p < 0.001$).

Table 4-13   Main internal reasons in different education levels

		Illiteracy (N=601)	Primary school (N=981)	Junior high school (N=1,381)	High school (N=775)	College and above (N=495)	χ^2	p
Hospital distance	No.	431	676	850	409	256	94.219	<0.001***
	%	71.70%	68.90%	61.50%	52.80%	51.70%		
	AR	5.3	5.1	-0.4	-5.8	-5		
Rational medical charge	No.	156	303	437	236	155	6.932	0.106
	%	26.00%	30.90%	31.60%	30.50%	31.30%		
	AR	-2.6	0.4	1.2	0	0.5		
Hospital staff service attitude	No.	108	175	333	201	115	26.596	<0.001***
	%	18.00%	17.80%	24.10%	25.90%	23.20%		
	AR	-2.6	-3.6	2.3	2.9	0.7		
Doctors' and nurses' professional skills	No.	83	160	285	234	152	96.568	<0.001***
	%	13.80%	16.30%	20.60%	30.20%	30.70%		
	AR	-5	-4.6	-1.1	6.4	5.2		

* $p<0.05$, ** $p<0.01$, *** $p<0.001$.

4.4　Discussion

Patients' health-seeking behavior analysis is an important and commonly used indicator for health care providers and payers to evaluate patients' health demand and medical service quality. Determinants of patients' choice of health care providers research also can provide scientific basis for the allocation of care resources. Although several empirical researches have been completed to analyze Chinese patients' health-seeking behavior, no intensive study has been performed to explore outpatients' choice of healthcare providers with large-sample evidence covering the backward provinces.

In the research, primary health care outpatients' health-seeking behavior of 11 provinces in rural western China were analyzed, a total of 4, 233 participants form 164 health care institutions completed the questionnaire, and the response rate was 91. 7%. Among all the respondents, 56. 8% were female, 46. 6% were farmers and 70. 9% were insured with the New Rural Cooperative Medical Scheme.

As presented Figure 4-2, according to China's National Health Service Survey (NHSS) report (2013), 57. 4% of Chinese rural outpatients for the common illness chose village clinics as the primary option to cure common illness, 23. 7% would visit township health centers, and 20% chose county and higher level hospitals. In this study, outpatients in rural western China were more likely to visit township health center and higher-level hospital, only 17. 6% of patients chose village clinics as primary health care provider. outpatients from township health centers and county hospitals who were studied in this research may have higher demand for health care and better disease recognition than outpatients who chose self-treatment. (Habtom & Ruys, 2007) It should also be noted that the overall patient health care demand may increase since the NHSS in 2013, for the growth of medical technology and individual socioeconomic status during the past few years. Therefore, it is reasonable that respondents in this research chose higher level institutions than the rural outpatients in the report.

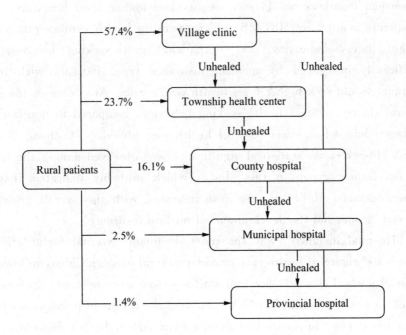

Figure 4-2　The heath-seeking pathways for
Chinese rural outpatients reported in NHSS (2013)

As previously reported, patient characteristics were the main internal determinants that influence patients' health-seeking behavior. Multinomial logistic regression results demonstrated that sample hospital type, province, gender, income, occupation, education level, medical insurance type and chronic disease condition were Statistically significant factors. Women interviewees inclined to visit higher level hospital, while male respondents were more likely to choose village clinics and township health centers, indicating that women and children may have greater demand of health care than adult men. This result was agreeable with the higher 2-week prevalence rate of women and children. Studies in other developing areas also showed similar conclusion. Outpatients with higher education and income level were more likely to select higher level hospitals, suggesting that patients with higher socioeconomic status have better disease recognition and greater demand of health care. The similar trend was also observed in China's urban areas. Compared with outpatients without medical insurance, respondents with urban insurance would visit county and higher level hospitals, while outpatients insured by NRCMS prefer township health centers rather than village clinics, indicating that outpatient health-seeking behavior was significantly influenced by medical insurance type. Patients with higher insurance would seek higher level health care service. According to the study of rural elderly resident health-seeking behavior, compared to non-farmers, farmers would select lower level of health care providers. (Zhang & Zou, 2014). However, no statistical significance was observed among the farmer and non-farmer group in this study, which probably indicated that the farmers' demand of health care have increased with the overall growth of personal income and the development of medical insurance.

"Hospital distance" was the most dominant external factor affecting outpatients' choice of health care provider in rural western China, followed by "rational medical charge" "hospital staff's service attitude" and "doctors' and nurses' professional skills", which supported the results of previous studies in urban areas. The Chi-square test p-values and ARs indicated that outpatients who chose higher level hospitals cared more about "doctors' and nurses' professional skills" and "hospital staff service attitude", and outpatients who selected village clinics cared more about "hospital distance", which showed that outpatients visit different hospitals with different expectations. And the association between patient characteristics and dominant external reasons demonstrated that the importance of "doctors' and nurses' professional skills" would increase with the promotion of socioeconomic status, while farmers, the elderly, male patients and residents with lower medical insurance cared more about "hospital distance". "Rational medical charge" "hospital staff service attitude" would gain more attention when outpatients were suffering from chronic diseases.

In this study, outpatients' medical choice was proved a complex of dimensional medical demand in different aspects, which were also affected by outpatient demographic characteristics, medical insurance coverage and disease severity. According to the research findings, outpatients from rural western China visited village clinics for convenience and timely service, and higher level hospitals for better service attitude and professional skills. Different aspects of service should be assessed, corresponding to patients' specific demands. Hierarchical medical treatment system also requests the diversity of health care. Village clinics and township health centers should improve accessibility of primary health care, county and higher-level hospitals should improve professional skills and service attitude, to ensure the affordability and satisfy patients' higher level of care demands. Different measures should be used to evaluate the service quality of different levels of hospitals, to encourage the efficient care delivery. Meanwhile, effort should be expended to develop overall health care service in backward regions, increase rural resident insurance coverage and illness recognition, ensure appropriate care, and promote the balanced allocation of care resources between urban and rural areas.

Chapter 5　Result Ⅱ:Outpatients' satisfaction in rural western China

The questionnaire survey was conducted from October to December 2014. A total of 4,616 patients participated in the survey, and 4,026 questionnaires were completed. The missing value rate for each item was 0.2% to 0.5%, and the total response rate was 87.2%, indicating that the questionnaire was acceptable and feasible.

5.1　Descriptive findings

The descriptive results of participants' demographic and other background characteristics are presented in Table 5-1. The mean age of respondents was 39.48 (SD=15.29); 56.9% were female, and 43.1% were male. Only 30.6% of the interviewees had completed high school or higher education. Farmer was the most common occupation, and 73.4% of responders' income were less than 2,001 *yuan* (about $330) per month. Most participants were enrolled in public medical insurance: 11.7% of respondents were insured by Urban Employee Basic Medical Insurance (UEBMI); 6.8% were insured by Urban Resident Basic Medical Insurance (URBMI), and 70.3% were insured by New Rural Cooperative Medical Scheme (NRCMS). About 1/4 of participants were suffering from chronic diseases.

Table 5-1　　　　　　　　　　**Respondents' characteristics**

Characteristics	No.	%
Gender		
Female	2,291	56.9

Continued

Characteristics	No.	%
Male	1,735	43.1
Education		
Illiteracy	560	13.9
Primary school	919	22.8
Junior high school	1316	32.7
High school	752	18.7
College or above	479	11.9
Occupation		
Farmer	1871	46.5
Blue-collar worker	443	11.0
Business/Service/Enterprise employee	563	14.0
Teacher/Government or public-sector staff	370	9.2
Student/Unemployed/Other jobs	697	17.3
Retirement	82	2.0
Monthly income		
Without income	1,073	26.7
1-2,000 *yuan*	1,881	46.7
2,001-4,000 *yuan*	848	21.1
4,001 *yuan* and more	224	5.6
Medical insurance		
National health insurance	109	2.7
UEBMI	473	11.7
URBMI	274	6.8
NRCMS	2,832	70.3
Medical insurance for urban and rural residents	93	2.3
Other insurances	52	1.3
No medical insurance	193	4.8
Chronic diseases		
Yes	1022	25.4
No	3,004	74.6

Table 5-2 shows the respondents' characteristics of different sample hospital levels. A total of 1,713 respondents were selected from township health centers, while 2,313 were selected from county-level hospitals. According to the Chi-square tests, statistical significances were also observed in the distribution of education level, occupation, monthly income, medical insurance type, and chronic disease conditions between township health centers and county-level hospitals, with all p values less than 0.001. The mean age of interviewees from township health centers were 42.44 (SD＝16.00), significantly older than the 37.28 (SD＝14.36) of county-level hospitals ($p <$ 0.001). And the proportion of female outpatients (60.4%) in county-level hospitals was higher than that of township health centers (52.2%, $p < 0.001$). Only 19.2% of the respondents from township health centers accepted high school or higher education, and high school achievement rate of outpatient from county-level hospitals was 39%. 60% participants from township health centers were farmers, while the proportion of farmers from county-level hospitals was 36.2%. 22% of outpatients from township health centers and 30% from county-level hospitals earned more than 2,001 *yuan* (about $ 330) per month, respectively. About 81% of respondents from township health centers were insured by New Rural Cooperative Medical Scheme (NRCMS), which was higher than the 62.0% of county-level hospitals. The chronic disease prevalence of participants from township health centers was 31.7%, which was high than the 20.7% of county-level hospitals.

Table 5-2　　　Respondents' characteristics, by sample hospital level

Characteristics	Township health centers N=1,713	County-level hospitals N=2,313
Mean age	42.44(±16.00)	37.28(±14.36)
Gender　($p < 0.001$***)		
Female	895(52.2%)	1,396(60.4%)
Male	818(47.8%)	917(39.6%)
Education　($p < 0.001$***)		
Illiteracy	319(18.6%)	241(10.4%)
Primary school	479(28.0%)	440(19.0%)

Continued

Characteristics	Township health centers N=1,713	County-level hospitals N=2,313
Junior high school	587(34.3%)	729(31.5%)
High school	222(13.0%)	530(22.9%)
College or above	106(6.2%)	373(16.1%)
Occupation ($p<0.001^{***}$)		
Farmer	1,033(60.3%)	838(36.2%)
Blue-collar worker	187(10.9%)	256(11.1%)
Business/Service/ Enterprise employee	166(9.7%)	397(17.2%)
Teacher/Governments or publicsector staff	103(6.0%)	267(11.5%)
Student/Unemployed/ Other jobs	192(11.2%)	505(21.8%)
Retirement	32(1.9%)	50(2.2%)
Monthly income ($p<0.001^{***}$)		
Without income	513(29.9%)	560(24.2%)
1-2,000 *yuan*	820(47.9%)	1,061(45.9%)
2,001-4,000 *yuan*	292(17.0%)	556(24.0%)
4,001 *yuan* and above	88(5.1%)	136(5.9%)
Medical insurance ($p<0.001^{***}$)		
National health insurance	28(1.6%)	81(3.5%)
UEBMI	119(6.9%)	354(15.3%)
URBMI	73(4.3%)	201(8.7%)
NRCMS	1,397(81.6%)	1,435(62.0%)
Medical insurance for urban and rural residents	34(2.0%)	59(2.6%)
Other insurances	17(1.0%)	35(1.5%)
No medical insurance	45(2.6%)	148(6.4%)

Continued

Characteristics	Township health centers N=1,713	County-level hospitals N=2,313
Chronic diseases　($p<0.001^{***}$)		
Yes	543(31.7%)	479(20.7%)
No	1,170(68.3%)	1,834(79.3%)

$^{*}p<0.05$，$^{**}p<0.01$，$^{***}p<0.001$.

5.2　Outpatients' satisfaction item scores

The results of the outpatients' satisfaction survey are shown in detail in Table 5-3.

The mean satisfaction item score of "time spent commuting to hospital" was 3.30 (SD=0.95), higher than the 3.14 (SD=0.97) of "waiting time". The mean score of "doctors' disease description" was 3.69. The mean score of "Patients' participation in decision-making" was 3.62 (SD=0.89). The mean score of "service attitude" was 3.75 (SD=0.86). The mean score of "hospital facility" was 3.32 (SD=0.83), lower than "hospital environment" (3.35 ± 0.82). The mean satisfaction score of "medical cost" was 3.16 (SD=0.87). The mean score of "doctors' and nurses' professional skills" was 3.61 (SD=0.75). The sum of mean scores of nine items was 30.94, with the maximum score of 45. According to the mean scores, respondents were satisfied with "service attitude" the most and then the "doctors' disease description". Waiting time was the least satisfactory item, followed by medical cost.

Table 5-3

Outpatients' satisfaction item scores

	Contents	Very dissatisfied	Dissatisfied	Neither satisfied nor dissatisfied	Satisfied	Very satisfied	Mean±SD
X_1	Time spent commuting to hospital	159(3.91%)	503(12.5%)	1,763(43.8%)	1186(29.5%)	415(10.3%)	3.30±0.95
X_2	Waiting time	206(5.1%)	678(16.8%)	1,852(46.0%)	939(23.3%)	351(8.7%)	3.14±0.97
X_3	Doctors' disease description	66(1.6%)	137(3.4%)	1,382(34.3%)	1,820(45.3%)	621(15.4%)	3.69±0.83
X_4	Patients' participation in decision-making	122(3.0%)	163(4.0%)	1,399(34.7%)	1,765(43.8%)	577(14.3%)	3.62±0.89
X_5	Service attitude	69(1.7%)	154(3.8%)	1,235(30.7%)	1,828(45.4%)	740(18.4%)	3.75±0.86
X_6	Hospital facility	81(2.0%)	390(9.7%)	2,050(50.9%)	1,178(29.3%)	327(8.1%)	3.32±0.83
X_7	Hospital environment	69(1.7%)	373(9.3%)	2,000(49.7%)	1,261(31.3%)	323(8.0%)	3.35±0.82
X_8	Medical cost	96(2.4%)	668(16.6%)	2,068(51.4%)	887(22.0%)	307(7.6%)	3.16±0.87
X_9	Doctors' and nurses' professional skills	31(0.8%)	143(3.6%)	1,584(39.3%)	1,863(46.3%)	405(10.1%)	3.61±0.75

The mean outpatient satisfaction item scores of respondents from township health centers and county-level hospitals were also analyzed, respectively.

As shown in Table 5-4, the t-test results indicates that outpatients from township health centers had significantly higher satisfaction scores in "time spent commuting to hospitals" ($p = 0.006$), "waiting time" ($p < 0.001$) and "medical cost" ($p < 0.001$) than county-level hospitals, and lower satisfaction scores in "hospital facility" ($p < 0.001$), "hospital environment" ($p < 0.001$) and "doctors' and nurses' professional skills" ($p = 0.003$). The mean item score of respondents from township health centers was 31.16, which was higher than the 30.77 of county-level hospitals.

Table 5-4   Mean outpatients' satisfaction item scores, by sample hospital levels

	Contents	Township health center Mean ($\pm$SD)	County-level hospitals Mean ($\pm$SD)	p
X_1	Time spent commuting to hospital	3.35($\pm$0.95)	3.26($\pm$0.95)	0.006**
X_2	Waiting time	3.26($\pm$0.97)	3.05($\pm$0.95)	<0.001***
X_3	Doctors' disease description	3.72($\pm$0.83)	3.67($\pm$0.83)	0.056
X_4	Patients' participation in decision-making	3.65($\pm$0.89)	3.61($\pm$0.89)	0.181
X_5	Service attitude	3.76($\pm$0.90)	3.74($\pm$0.82)	0.564
X_6	Hospital facility	3.16($\pm$0.83)	3.43($\pm$0.81)	<0.001***
X_7	Hospital environment	3.29($\pm$0.81)	3.39($\pm$0.83)	<0.001***
X_8	Medical cost	3.40($\pm$0.88)	2.98($\pm$0.82)	<0.001***

* $p < 0.05$, ** $p < 0.01$, *** $p < 0.001$.

Significant differences were observed of the mean satisfaction item scores of "waiting time" ($p < 0.001$), "service attitude" ($p = 0.007$), "hospital facility" ($p = 0.035$) and "hospital environment" ($p = 0.039$) among different county-level hospitals. Outpatients from county-hospitals of TCM had the highest scores of "waiting time" (3.20 ± 0.92) and "service attitude" (3.82 ± 0.76). However, participants from county general hospitals had the highest scores of "hospital facility" (3.48 ± 0.87) and "hospital environment" (3.44 ± 0.88). The mean item score of outpatients from county general hospitals was 30.76, which was higher than the 30.58 of county MCHs, but lower than the 30.97 of county hospitals of TCM. See details in Table 5-5 and Figure 5-1.

Table 5-5   Satisfaction item scores, by county-level hospitals

	Contents	County general hospitals Mean ($\pm$SD)	County MCHs Mean ($\pm$SD)	County hospitals of TCM Mean ($\pm$SD)	p
X_1	Time spent commuting to hospital	3.23($\pm$1.00)	3.25($\pm$0.92)	3.32($\pm$0.89)	0.121
X_2	Waiting time	3.00($\pm$1.00)	2.95($\pm$0.89)	3.20($\pm$0.92)	<0.001***
X_3	Doctors' disease description	3.68($\pm$0.88)	3.66($\pm$0.78)	3.68($\pm$0.80)	0.860
X_4	Patients' participation in decision-making	3.59($\pm$0.94)	3.61($\pm$0.84)	3.63($\pm$0.85)	0.547
X_5	Service attitude	3.73($\pm$0.86)	3.69($\pm$0.81)	3.82($\pm$0.76)	0.007**
X_6	Hospital facility	3.48($\pm$0.87)	3.41($\pm$0.79)	3.38($\pm$0.74)	0.035*
X_7	Hospital environment	3.44($\pm$0.88)	3.36($\pm$0.78)	3.34($\pm$0.78)	0.039*
X_8	Medical cost	2.98($\pm$0.83)	3.00($\pm$0.83)	2.96($\pm$0.82)	0.683
X_9	Doctors' and nurses' professional skills	3.64($\pm$0.78)	3.66($\pm$0.69)	3.64($\pm$0.72)	0.835

* $p<0.05$, ** $p<0.01$, *** $p<0.001$.

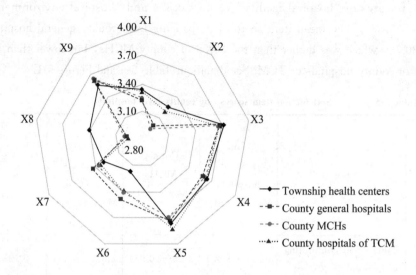

Figure 5-1　Satisfaction item scores, by sample hospitals

5.3　Factor analysis

Exploratory factor analysis was conducted to explore the dimensionality of the overall outpatients' satisfaction in rural western China, and to analyze the validity of the dimensional structure.

The overall Cronbach's alpha value was 0.73, suggesting good reliability. The KMO measure for the data set was 0.777, the Bartlett's test was 7496.478 ($p < 0.001$), and all MSAvalues exceeded 0.50, implying that the data was adequate for EFA. (Field, 2013; Pallant, 2013; Wu, 2010) The communalities of each item (h^2) are demonstrated in Table 5-6.

Table 5-6　　　　　　　　　　　**Communalities**

	Contents	Initial	Extraction
X_1	Time spent commuting to hospital	1.000	0.619
X_2	Waiting time	1.000	0.655
X_3	Doctors' disease description	1.000	0.710

Continued

	Contents	Initial	Extraction
X_4	Patients' participation in decision-making	1.000	0.716
X_5	Service attitude	1.000	0.465
X_6	Hospital facility	1.000	0.723
X_7	Hospital environment	1.000	0.696
X_8	Medical cost	1.000	0.360
X_9	Doctors' and nurses' professional skills	1.000	0.512

Principal component analysis and varimax rotation were adopted. As shown in Table 5-7, only two factors had eigenvalues greater than 1. However, with the combination of the cumulative variance percentage and scree plot (see Figure 1-5-2), a 3-factor solution was applied in the factor analysis.

Table 5-7　　　　　**Factor eigenvalues and variance percentage**

Components	Initial eigenvalue			Rotation sums of square loadings		
	Total	% of variance	Cumulative %	Total	% of variance	Cumulative %
1	2.970	33.002	33.002	1.923	21.372	21.372
2	1.578	17.533	50.535	1.810	20.108	41.480
3	0.907	10.076	60.611	1.722	19.131	60.611
4	0.833	9.255	69.866			
5	0.662	7.360	77.225			
6	0.611	6.791	84.016			
7	0.549	6.096	90.112			
8	0.474	5.265	95.377			
9	0.416	4.623	100.000			

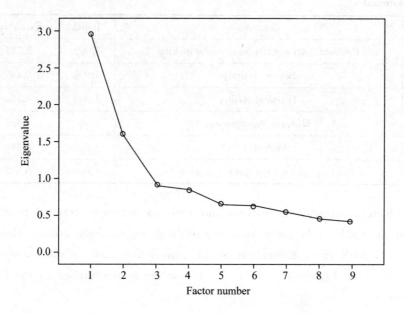

Figure 5-2　Scree plot

The correlation between the variables and the factor were shown in Table 5-8 and Table 5-9, which also presented the rotated factor loadings.

According to the factor loading values, nine items were explained by three dimensions. Factor 1 "service attitude" consisted of three items of the questionnaire, including "patients' participation in decision-making" "doctors' disease description", and "service attitude", accounting for 21.372% of variance. Factor 2 "facility and professional skills" consisted of "hospital environment" "hospital facility" and "doctors' and nurses' professional skills", explaining 20.108% of variance. Factor 3 "patients' cost" consisted of three items, including "waiting time" "time spent commuting to hospital", and "medical cost", and contributed 19.131% of variance.

Table 5-8　　　　　　　　　　　　　　Factor matrix[a]

		Factors		
		1	2	3
X_1	Time spent commuting to hospital	0.233	0.688	0.301
X_2	Waiting time	0.346	0.728	0.071

Continued

		Factors		
		1	2	3
X_3	Doctors' disease description	0.728	−0.142	−0.400
X_4	Patients' participation in decision-making	0.702	−0.129	−0.454
X_5	Service attitude	0.627	0.233	−0.133
X_6	Hospital facility	0.630	−0.378	0.427
X_7	Hospital environment	0.640	−0.244	0.476
X_8	Medical cost	0.326	0.494	−0.101
X_9	Doctors' and nurses' professional skills	0.685	−0.189	0.085

Extraction Method: Principal Axis Factoring

a.3 factors extracted

Table 5-9   **Rotated factor matrix[a]**

		Factors		
		1	2	3
X_1	Time spent commuting to hospital	−0.135	0.099	0.769
X_2	Waiting time	0.101	−0.003	0.803
X_3	Doctors' disease description	0.808	0.234	0.048
X_4	Patients' participation in decision-making	0.826	0.176	0.041
X_5	Service attitude	0.503	0.216	0.406
X_6	Hospital facility	0.186	0.828	−0.055
X_7	Hospital environment	0.141	0.818	0.081
X_8	Medical cost	0.237	−0.047	0.549
X_9	Doctors' and nurses' professional skills	0.442	0.558	0.078

Extraction Method: Principal Axis Factoring

Rotation Method: Varimax with Kaisa Normalization

a.Rotation converged in 5 iterations

The internal consistency of the matrix was examined (Table 5-10). For Factor 1 and Factor 2, the Cronbach's alpha value were 0.687 and 0.696 respectively, which showed good reliability. The inter item correlation (IIC) can also be adopted as a measure of internal consistency when the number of items in the scale was less than 10, which was acceptable between 0.2 and 0.4. Thus, the internal consistency of Factor 3 was considered acceptable though the Cronbach's alpha value was only 0.556.

Table 5-10   Factor structure and the internal consistency

	Factors and contents	Loadings	Cronbach's Alpha	IIC
	Service attitude (Factor 1)		0.687	0.422
X_4	Patients' participation in decision-making	0.769		
X_3	Doctors' disease description	0.808		
X_5	Service attitude	0.503		
	Facility and professional skills (Factor2)		0.696	0.432
X_7	Hospital environment	0.818		
X_6	Hospital facility	0.828		
X_9	Doctors' and nurses' professional skills	0.558		
	Patients' cost (Factor 3)		0.556	0.294
X_2	Waiting time	0.803		
X_1	Time spent commuting to hospital	0.769		
X_8	Medical cost	0.549		

5.4 Determinants of outpatients' satisfaction

The regression method was used to estimate the factor score coefficients (see Table 5-11), and the scores of Factor 1 (F_1), Factor 2 (F_2) and Factor 3 (F_3) were produced by SPSS software. In order to comprehensively explore the characteristics associated with outpatients' satisfaction, the factor score of overall satisfaction (F) was calculated based on the score and variance contribution rate of the three main factors as follows:

$$F = 0.21372 \ F_1 + 0.20108 \ F_2 + 0.19131 \ F_3$$

Table 5-11   **Factor score coefficient matrix**

		Factors		
		1	2	3
X_1	Time spent commuting to hospital	−0.234	0.116	0.489
X_2	Waiting time	−0.031	−0.044	0.479
X_3	Doctors' disease description	0.493	−0.116	−0.078
X_4	Patients' participation in decision-making	0.528	−0.165	−0.084
X_5	Service attitude	0.233	−0.023	0.182
X_6	Hospital facility	−0.154	0.544	−0.063
X_7	Hospital environment	−0.201	0.553	0.026
X_8	Medical cost	0.116	−0.123	0.306
X_9	Doctors' and nurses' professional skills	0.110	0.253	−0.014

Extraction Method: Principal Axis Factoring

Rotation Method: Varimax with Kaisa Normalization

Stepwise multiple linear regression was conducted to investigate the factors associated with the three main dimensions and the overall satisfaction. Patients' age, sample hospital type, education, occupation, monthly income, medical insurance type and chronic disease condition showed significant differences in the univariate analysis (See details in Table 5-12 to Table 5-18), and thus were included in regression model as independent variables, with F_1, F_2, F_3 and F as dependent variables, respectively.

Table 5-12   **Association between outpatients' satisfaction and age**

	Age	
	Pearson correlation	p
Service attitude (F_1)	0.002	0.170
Facility and professional skills (F_2)	−0.018	0.251
Patients' cost (F_3)	0.126	<0.001***
Overall satisfaction (F)	0.072	<0.001***

* $p<0.05$, ** $p<0.01$, *** $p<0.001$.

Table 5-13　　　　　**Outpatients' satisfaction in different hospitals**

	Sample hospital type				
	Township health center	County general hospital	County MCH	County hospital of TCM	p
Service attitude (F_1)	0.085	−0.090	−0.061	−0.023	<0.001***
Facility and professional skills (F_2)	−0.193	0.206	0.117	0.069	<0.001***
Patients' cost (F_3)	0.178	−0.172	−0.190	−0.016	<0.001***
Overall satisfaction (F)	0.013	−0.011	−0.026	0.006	0.063

* $p<0.05$, ** $p<0.01$, *** $p<0.001$.

Table 5-14　　　　　**Outpatients' satisfaction in different education levels**

	Education					
	Illiteracy	Primary school	Junior high school	High school	College or above	p
Service attitude (F_1)	−0.105	−0.088	0.018	0.104	0.080	<0.001***
Facility and professional skills (F_2)	−0.040	−0.107	−0.004	0.046	0.191	<0.001***
Patients' cost (F_3)	0.199	0.107	−0.028	−0.132	−0.154	<0.001***
Overall satisfaction (F)	0.008	−0.020	−0.002	0.006	0.026	0.177

* $p<0.05$, ** $p<0.01$, *** $p<0.001$.

Table 5-15　　　Outpatient satisfaction in different occupations

	Occupation						
	Farmer	Worker	Business/ Service/ Enterprise employee	Teacher/ Government staff	Student/ Unemployment/ Others	Retirement	p
F_1	0.053	−0.111	0.000	0.140	−0.176	0.257	<0.001***
F_2	−0.041	−0.099	0.037	0.125	0.068	0.085	0.004**
F_3	0.092	−0.062	−0.120	−0.036	−0.108	0.137	<0.001***
F	0.021	−0.055	−0.015	0.048	−0.045	0.098	<0.001***

* $p<0.05$, ** $p<0.01$, *** $p<0.001$.

able 5-16　　　Outpatient satisfaction in different income levels

	Monthly income (RMB)				
	Without income	1-2,000 *yuan*	2,001-4,000 *yuan*	⩾4,001 *yuan*	p
Service attitude (F_1)	0.023	−0.013	−0.002	0.007	0.825
Facility and professional skills (F_2)	−0.063	0.013	0.021	0.111	0.068
Patients' cost (F_3)	−0.068	0.060	−0.014	−0.128	0.001**
Overall satisfaction (F)	−0.021	0.011	0.001	−0.001	0.128

* $p<0.05$, ** $p<0.01$, *** $p<0.001$.

Table 5-17　　　Outpatient satisfaction in different insurance types

	Medical insurance type							
	National health insurance	UEBMI	URBMI	NRCMS	Medical insurance for urban and rural residents	Other insurances	No insurance	p
F_1	0.195	0.088	−0.049	−0.008	−0.046	−0.103	−0.095	0.097
F_2	0.284	0.088	0.123	−0.042	−0.075	0.044	0.085	0.001**
F_3	−0.165	−0.038	−0.190	0.057	−0.020	−0.467	−0.242	<0.001***
F	0.067	0.029	−0.022	0.001	−0.029	−0.102	−0.050	0.013**

* $p<0.05$, ** $p<0.01$, *** $p<0.001$.

Table 5-18　Outpatients' satisfaction in different chronic disease conditions

	Chronic disease conditions		
	With chronic disease	Without chronic disease	p
Service attitude (F_1)	0.162	−0.055	<0.001***
Facility and professional skills (F_2)	0.087	−0.030	<0.001***
Patients' cost (F_3)	−0.018	0.006	0.524
Overall satisfaction (F)	0.049	0.017	<0.001***

*$p<0.05$，**$p<0.01$，***$p<0.001$.

Table 5-19 presents the results of the stepwise multiple linear regression, which demonstrates that the age, sample hospital type, education, occupation, medical insurance type, monthly income and chronic disease condition were statistically associated with the dimensional or overall outpatients' satisfaction.

According to the coefficients and p values, significant differences were observed among different respondent populations in dimensional satisfaction: older outpatients had higher satisfaction score in "patients' cost"; interviewees from county-level hospitals were more satisfied with "facility and professional skills", but less satisfied with the other two dimensions than township health centers; compared to lower educated patients, respondents with junior middle school and higher education were more satisfied with "service attitude" and "facility and professional skills", less satisfied with "patients' cost"; farmers, in comparison with other patients, were more satisfied with "service attitude"; respondents insured by national health insurance and UEBMI were more satisfied with "service attitude" than other outpatients; higher income participants were more satisfied with "patients' cost"; outpatients with chronic diseases were more satisfied with "service attitude" and "facility and professional skills", but less with "patients' cost".

Different respondents also had significant differences in overall satisfaction: the overall satisfaction increased significantly with age; higher educated respondents were more satisfied; compared with other occupations, farmers were more satisfied with overall outpatient health care; respondents insured by national health insurance and UEBMI were more satisfied than other outpatients; respondents with chronic diseases had higher overall satisfaction.

Table 5-19

Determinants of outpatients' satisfaction

Variable	Service attitude (F_1)		Facility and professional skills (F_2)		Patients' cost (F_3)		Overall satisfaction (F)	
	β	p	β	p	β	p	β	p
Age					0.006	<0.001***	0.001	<0.001***
Sample hospital type								
Township health centers[a]								
Other county hospitals	−0.112	0.003**	0.293	<0.001***	−0.319	<0.001***		
County general hospitals	−0.175	<0.001***	0.396	<0.001***	−0.238	<0.001***		
Education								
Primary school or less[a]								
Junior middle school or higher	0.238	<0.001***	0.086	0.009**	−0.128	<0.001***	0.046	<0.001***
Occupation								
Others[a]								
Farmers	0.238	<0.001***					0.051	<0.001***
Medical insurance type								
Others[a]								
National health insurance/UEBMI	0.147	0.002**					0.045	0.009**
Monthly income								
Without income[a]								

西部农村居民对医疗服务的认知：
基于消费者决策过程理论的实证研究

Continued

Variable	Service attitude (F₁) β	p	Facility and professional skills (F₂) β	p	Patients' cost (F₃) β	p	Overall satisfaction (F) β	P
1-2,000 *yuan*					0.143	<0.001***	0.047	0.014*
2,001 *yuan* and more					0.122	0.006**	0.024	0.157
Chronic diseases								
No[a]								
Yes	0.203	<0.001***	0.175	<0.001***	−0.131	<0.001***	0.053	0.002**

* $p<0.05$, ** $p<0.01$, *** $p<0.001$.
a: Reference category

5.5 Discussion

Patients' satisfaction is an important and commonly used indicator to analyze the patients demand, performance and utilization of medical service. Therefore, patients' satisfaction research is essential in the process of China's health system reform. Although several patient satisfaction reports had been published before, no intensive study was conducted to investigate outpatients' satisfaction with large sample evidence covering China's backward provinces.

In this research, primary health care outpatients' satisfaction of 11 provinces in western China were analyzed. A total of 4,026 outpatients completed the questionnaire, among which 1,713 respondents were selected from township health centers, while 2,313 from county-level hospitals. The questionnaire response rate was 87.2%. For all the respondents, 46.5% were farmers and 70.3% were insured with the New Rural Cooperative Medical Scheme.

EFA results showed a three-dimension structure of overall outpatients' satisfaction, "service attitude" "facility and professional skills" and "patients' cost" with 3 items, respectively, and demonstrated acceptable reliability and validity. Each factor accounted for about 20% of variance. The stepwise multiple linear regression results indicated that age, sample hospital type, education, occupation, medical insurance type, monthly income and chronic disease condition were statistically associated with dimensional or overall outpatients' satisfaction.

The overall satisfaction increased with age, which was agreeable to the report of outpatients' satisfaction in Ningxia and Shanghai. Respondents with chronic diseases tended to have higher overall satisfaction, and the similar trend was observed in satisfaction study from developed areas. (Bao et al., 2015) It was possible that the elderly and chronic patients, compared with the young and patients without chronic diseases, were more experienced and trust their doctors due to the health status. Participants from county-level general hospital were less satisfied with "patients' cost" than other hospitals, because "waiting time" was reported as the most important item of patient satisfaction in general hospitals. (Yuan & Li, 2015) This result may suggest that outpatients in county-level hospitals requested more efficient care service. Outpatients with higher income were more satisfied with "patient cost", predicting that the economic burden would be relieved with the increasing income of Chinese residents. Contrary to the previous evidence (Zhou, Mei, Zhang & Shao, 2011), though less satisfied with "patients' cost", better educated outpatients were more satisfied with "service attitude" "facility and professional skills". It was probable the accessibility to high-quality medical service rather than the affordability that influenced the overall satisfaction of educated outpatients in rural western China. Outpatients insured by national health insurance and UEBMI were more satisfied with "service attitude" and overall outpatient service, which may be related with the higher insurance coverage. Compared with other occupations, farmers had higher "service attitude" satisfaction and overall satisfaction, while no significant difference was observed in satisfaction of "patient cost", indicating that with the growth of socio-economic status of farmers, "service attitude" may be the most dominant dimension of outpatient health care.

Patient satisfaction is a reflection of residents' health care demands, so that understanding the demand of patients under different conditions plays a crucial role in improving the performance and efficiency of medical services. There are similarities and differences between the results in this survey and previous studies, which suggests that outpatients' health care demands in rural western China have their own uniqueness. However, considering the association between outpatients' characteristics and satisfaction in this study, primary demands of some rural outpatients have altered from lower price to higher efficiency, better service attitude and professional skills. Since China has implemented the National Essential Medicines List in 2009 and required no drug profit margins in public hospitals in 2017, a universal access to affordable essential medicines would be gotten in a few years. Healthcare providers should identify and target more initiatives to improve service attitude, environment and professional skills. In rural western China, efficient hospital management methods, modern technologies and more staff training are needed to improve the healthcare service quality. Implementation of electronic patient record system and consultation desk in each department may reduce the patients' queue time and doctors' preparation time in general hospitals. (Middleton et al., 2013) More interpersonal communication training would help doctors and nurses in disease explanation and promote service attitude. Rural primary health care institutions are also suggested to provide more patient education about chronic diseases, to promote patient participation and improve the care efficiency. (Nie, Wu, Wang & Yuan, 2018)

Most published satisfaction questionnaire survey on Chinese patients were single-center study in tertiary hospitals or developed regions, conducting regression analysis on mean satisfaction score (Yu et al., 2016) or satisfaction rate (Zhou et al., 2011). Compared with previous studies, a questionnaire was developed in this study to collect primary health care outpatients' satisfaction score in rural western China. Then exploratory factor analysis and multilinear regression were conducted to describe the satisfaction dimension and associated factors, exploring rural outpatients' satisfaction from another perspective. It is the first outpatients' satisfaction questionnaire study based on EFA with multi-province evidence in backward China, and the questionnaire shows acceptable reliability and good feasibility.

Chapter 6   Conclusion

This research is the first outpatients' perception questionnaire survey conducted in backward China with multi-center evidence from various provinces, exploring outpatients' choices of care providers and satisfaction of the service, on the basis of consumer decision process theory.

This survey investigates outpatient choice of care provider of common illness in rural western China, analyzes the internal and external determinants associated with outpatient health seeking behavior. According to the results, township health center was the primary option for nearly half of the responders, outpatients with better socioeconomic status cared more about "doctors' and nurses' professional skills" and "service attitude", and tended to select higher level hospitals; outpatients who chose village clinics cared more about "hospital distance". And the results also suggest that women and children may have greater demands of health care than adult men.

The primary health care outpatient satisfaction in rural western China was lower than developed areas and tertiary hospitals, "service attitude" "facility and professional skills" and "patients' cost" were the main three dimensions of overall satisfaction, with significant differences among patients with difference demographic characteristics and chronic disease conditions. With the growth of personal income and promotion of universal coverage, the dominant factor in outpatient evaluation would change from the affordability to the accessibility of high-quality care.

On the whole, there are similarities and differences between the results in this research and previous studies, suggesting that outpatients' perception and demand of health care in rural western China have their own features.

Different hospitals should fulfill different functions. The health care performance in rural western China is certainly needed to be improved.

6.1 Policy recommendations

According to the research results, the convenient and timely service of village clinics is preferred when outpatients from rural western China seek for primary health care services, and service attitude and professional skills are essential when visiting higher-level hospitals. Local health care providers should assess and manage the outpatient service quality based on the actual needs of patients, considering patients' demographic characteristics and health status. However, policy makers and care payers should evaluate the service performance of different hospitals based on different standards. Meanwhile, overall service quality, resident insurance coverage rate and illness recognition in backward regions need to be promoted, to ensure efficient health care delivery and impartial allocation of care resources.

In backward areas, efficient hospital management methods, modern technologies and staff trainings are still needed. The electronic patient record system and consultation desk in each department should be introduced in general hospitals, to reduce the patient queue time and doctor preparation time. Regular training sessions such as interpersonal communication would help doctors and nurses in disease explanation and promoting service attitude. Patient education about chronic disease management in rural primary health care institutions are also needed, to promote patient participation and improve the care efficiency.

6.2 Limitations

It should be noted that this study has some limitations:

Firstly, only outpatients from township health centers and county hospitals were interviewed in this research; the health-seeking behavior of rural residents who chose self-treatment cannot be analyzed from this study.

Secondly, the research sampling was not conducted based on the population distribution of 11 provinces, which may cause the deviation of sample resource.

Thirdly, residents of ethnic minorities may have their own ethnic doctors and medicine, and the health-seeking behavior of different ethnics need to be explored.

Fourthly, disparities of economic level and medical service quality among 11 provinces were not studied, so different patients' perception caused by them could not be explained in this study.

6.3 Perspectives for future work

This study focuses on the outpatients' perception of health care service from rural western China, but outpatients' perception from rural areas in developed areas or eastern China could also be analyzed, and the disparity of patient health seeking behavior and preference between rural western China and rural eastern China can be studied. Given that only outpatients from township health centers and county hospitals were interviewed in this research, the health-seeking behavior of patients from village clinics and rural residents who chose self-treatment are still needed to be disclosed. Besides, the health-seeking behavior of different ethnic minorities can also be investigated in the future.

References

Agarwal, A., Sethi, A., Sareen, D. et al. (2011). Treatment delay in oral and oropharyngeal cancer in our population: the role of socio-economic factors and health-seeking behaviour. *Indian Journal of Otolaryngology and Head & Neck Surgery*, 63(2).

Agresti, A. (2013). *Categorical data analysis*. New York: John Wiley & Sons.

Aharony, L. & Strasser, S. (1993). Patient satisfaction: what we know about and what we still need to explore. *Medical Care Review*, 50(1).

Ahmed, S. M., Adams, A. M., Chowdhury, M. et al. (2000). Gender, socioeconomic development and health-seeking behaviour in Bangladesh. *Social Science & Medicine*, 51(3).

Al-Abri, R. & Al-Balushi, A. (2014). Patient satisfaction survey as a tool towards quality improvement. *Oman Medical Journal*, 29(1).

Andaleeb, S. S. (2001). Service quality perceptions and patient satisfaction: a study of hospitals in a developing country. *Social Science & Medicine*, 52(9).

Anhang P. R., Elliott, M. N., Zaslavsky, A. M. et al. (2014). Examining the role of patient experience surveys in measuring health care quality. *Medical Care Research and Review*, 71(5).

Assael, H. (1984). *Consumer behavior and marketing action*. Boston: Kent Pub. Co.

Bao, C., Zhou, Y., Li, J. et al. (2015). Investigation and analysis of outpatients' satisfaction of 2170 cases. *Chinese Hospital Management*, 35(9).

Batbaatar, E., Dorjdagva, J., Luvsannyam, A. et al. (2015).

Conceptualisation of patient satisfaction: a systematic narrative literature review. *Perspectives in Public Health*, 135(5).

Birk, H. O., Gut, R. & Henriksen, L. O. (2011). Patients'experience of choosing an outpatient clinic in one county in Denmark: results of a patient survey. *BMC Health Services Research*, 11(1).

Blackwell, R. D., Miniard, P. W. & Engel, J. F. (2006). *Consumer behavior*. Mason: Thomson/South-Western.

Blumenthal, D. & Hsiao, W. (2015). Lessons from the East—China's rapidly evolving health care system. *New England Journal of Medicine*, 372(14).

Boachie, M. K. (2016). Preferred primary healthcare provider choice among insured persons in Ashanti Region, Ghana. *International Journal of Health Policy and Management*, 5(3), 155.

Briggs, S. R. & Cheek, J. M. (1986). The role of factor analysis in the development and evaluation of personality scales. *Journal of Personality*, 54(1).

Brown, P. H. & Theoharides, C. (2009a). Health-seeking behavior and hospital choice in China's New Cooperative Medical System. *Health Economics*, 18(S2).

Brown, P. H. & Theoharides, C. (2009b). Health-seeking behavior and hospital choice in China's New Cooperative Medical System. *Health Economics*, 18(S2).

Cai, F. (2012). Is there a "Middle-income trap"? theories, experiences and relevance to China. *China & World Economy*, 20(1).

Cai, S., Cai, W., Deng, L. et al. (2016). Hospital organizational environment and staff satisfaction in China: A large-scale survey. *International Journal of Nursing Practice*, 22(6).

Cattell, R. B. (1966). The scree test for the number of factors. *Multivariate Behavioral Research*, 1(2).

Chen, A., Xu, A. & Zhang, G. (2017). Influencing factors of residents' choice of health care provider under the hierarchical medical system. *Chinese Journal of Health Statistics*, 34(5).

Chen, W., Tang, S., Sun, J. et al. (2010). Availability and use of essential medicines in China: manufacturing, supply, and prescribing in Shandong and Gansu provinces. *BMC Health Services Research*, 10(1).

Chen, X. (2012). Satisfaction study on rural community health care service in backward area. *Labor Security World*, (10).

Cheng, T. -M. (2012). Early results of China's historic health reforms: the view from Minister Chen Zhu. *Health Affairs*, 31(11).

Choi, K. -S., Cho, W.- H., Lee, S. et al. (2004). The relationships among quality, value, satisfaction and behavioral intention in health care provider choice: a South Korean study. *Journal of Business Research*, 57(8).

Chrisman, N. J. (1977). The health seeking process: an approach to the natural history of illness. *Culture, Medicine and Psychiatry*, 1(4).

Crow, R., Gage, H., Hampson, S. et al. (2002). Measurement of satisfaction with health care: implications for practice from a systematic review of the literature. *Health Technology Assessment*, 6(32).

DiClemente, C. C. & Prochaska, J. O. (1982). Self-change and therapy change of smoking behavior: a comparison of processes of change in cessation and maintenance. *Addictive Behaviors*, 7(2).

DiStefano, C., Zhu, M. & Mindrila, D. (2009). Understanding and using factor scores: considerations for the applied researcher. *Practical Assessment, Research & Evaluation*, 14(20).

Donabedian, A. (1980). *The definition of quality and approaches to its assessment*. Vol 1. *Explorations in quality assessment and monitoring*. Ann Arbor: Health Administration Press.

Duan, Z., Pan, J., Ren, Y. et al. (2016). Investigation and countermeasures of medical behavior of urban residents in Sichuan province. *Chinese Health Quality Management*, 1.

Eriksen, L. R. (1995). Patient satisfaction with nursing care: concept clarification. *Journal of Nursing Measurement*, 3(1).

Etier, B. E., Jr., Orr, S. P., Antonetti, J. et al. (2016). Factors impacting Press Ganey patient satisfaction scores in orthopedic surgery spine clinic. *The Spine Journal*, 16(11).

Field, A. (2013). *Discovering statistics using IBM SPSS statistics*. London: Sage Publications.

Fishbein, M. E. (1967). *Readings in attitude theory and measurement*. New York: John Wiley & Sons.

Fitzpatrick, R. & Hopkins, A. (1983). Problems in the conceptual framework of patient satisfaction research: an empirical exploration.

Sociology of Health & Illness, 5(3).

Fox, J. G. & Storms, D. M. (1981). A different approach to sociodemographic predictors of satisfaction with health care. *Social Science & Medicine. Part A: Medical Psychology & Medical Sociology*, 15(5).

Fung, C. H., Elliott, M. N., Hays, R. D. et al. (2005). Patients' preferences for technical versus interpersonal ability when selecting a primary care physician. *Health Services Research*, 40(4).

Garratt, A. M., Bjaertnes, O. A., Krogstad, U. et al. (2005). The outpatient experiences questionnaire (OPEQ): data quality, reliability, and validity in patients attending 52 Norwegian hospitals. *Quality & Safety in Health Care*, 14(6).

Ge, Z., Huang, J., Wang, M. et al. (2011). Analyzing the outpatients'satisfaction in township health clinics. *The Chinese Health Service Management*, 2.

Gill, L. & White, L. (2009). A critical review of patient satisfaction. *Leadership in Health Services*, 22(1).

Glanz, K., Rimer, B. K. & Viswanath, K. (2008). *Health behavior and health education: theory, research, and practice*. New York: John Wiley & Sons.

Goel, S., Sharma, D. & Singh, A. (2014). Development and validation of a patient satisfaction questionnaire for outpatients attending health centres in North Indian cities. *Journal of Health Services Research & Policy*, 19(2).

Grossman, M. (1972). On the concept of health capital and the demand for health. *Journal of Political Economy*, 80(2).

Grundy, J. & Annear, P. (2010). Health-seeking behavior studies: a literature review of study design and methods with a focus on Cambodia. *Health Policy and Health Finance Knowledge Hub Working Paper Series*, 7.

Haberman, S. J. (1973). The analysis of residuals in cross-classified tables. *Biometrics*, 29(1).

Habtom, G. K. & Ruys, P. (2007). The choice of a health care provider in Eritrea. *Health Policy*, 80(1).

Hampshire, K. R., Porter, G., Owusu, S. A. et al. (2011). Out of the reach of children? Young people's health-seeking practices and agency in Africa's newly-emerging therapeutic landscapes. *Social Science & Medicine*, 73(5).

Heidegger, T., Saal, D. & Nuebling, M. (2006). Patient satisfaction with anaesthesia care: what is patient satisfaction, how should it be measured, and what is the evidence for assuring high patient satisfaction? *Best Practice & Research Clinical Anaesthesiology*, 20(2).

Hills, R. & Kitchen, S. (2007). Development of a model of patient satisfaction with physiotherapy. *Physiotherapy Theory and Practice*, 23(5).

Hochbaum, G. M. (1958). Public participation in medical screening programs: a socio-psychological study. US Department of Health, Education, and Welfare, Public Health Service, Bureau of State Services, Division of Special Health Services, Tuberculosis Program.

Horn, J. L. (1965). A rationale and test for the number of factors in factor analysis. *Psychometrika*, 30.

Hosmer Jr, D. W., Lemeshow, S. & Sturdivant, R. X. (2013). *Applied logistic regression* (Vol. 398). New York: John Wiley & Sons.

Howard, J. A. & Sheth, J. N. (1969). *The theory of buyer behavior*. New York: John Wiley & Sons.

Hsiao, W. C. (2004). Disparity in health: the underbelly of China's economic development. *Harvard China Review*, 5(1).

Hu, S., Tang, S., Liu, Y. et al. (2008). Reform of how health care is paid for in China: challenges and opportunities. *The Lancet*, 372(9652).

Huang, F. & Gan, L. (2017). The impacts of China's urban employee basic medical insurance on healthcare expenditures and health outcomes. *Health Economics*, 26(2).

Hulka, B. S., Zyzanski, S. J., Cassel, J. C. et al. (1970). Scale for the measurement of attitudes toward physicians and primary medical care. *Medical Care*, 8(5).

Hunt, H. K., Institute, M. S. & Foundation, N. S. (1977). *Conceptualization and measurement of consumer satisfaction and dissatisfaction*. Cambridge, Mass: Marketing Science Institute.

Isaac, T., Zaslavsky, A. M., Cleary, P. D. et al. (2010). The relationship between patients' perception of care and measures of hospital quality and safety. *Health Services Research*, 45(4).

Jackson, M. D., Coombs, M. P., Wright, B. E. et al. (2004). Self-reported non-communicable chronic diseases and health-seeking behaviour in rural Jamaica, following a health promotion intervention: a preliminary report. Paper presented at the International Congress Series.

Janis, I. L. & Mann, L. (1979). *Decision making: a psychological analysis of conflict, choice, and commitment*. New York: Free Press.

Jaturapatporn, D., Hathirat, S., Manataweewat, B. et al. (2006). Reliability and validity of a Thai version of the General Practice Assessment Questionnaire (GPAQ). *Journal of the Medical Association of Thailand*, 89(9).

Jha, A. K., Orav, E. J., Zheng, J. et al. (2008). Patients' perception of hospital care in the United States. *New England Journal of Medicine*, 359(18).

Kaiser, H. F. (1960). The application of electronic computers to factor analysis. *Educational and Psychological Measurement*, 20(1).

Khamis, K. & Njau, B. (2014). Patients' level of satisfaction on quality of health care at Mwananyamala hospital in Dar es Salaam, Tanzania. *BMC Health Services Research*, 14(1).

Kleefstra, S. M., Kool, R. B., Veldkamp, C. M. et al. (2010). A core questionnaire for the assessment of patient satisfaction in academic hospitals in the Netherlands: development and first results in a nationwide study. *Quality & Safety in Health Care*, 19(5).

Kleefstra, S. M., Kool, R. B., Zandbelt, L. C. et al. (2012). An instrument assessing patient satisfaction with day care in hospitals. *BMC Health Services Research*, 12.

Kotler, P., Keller, K. L., Brady, M. et al. (2016). *Marketing Management*. London: Pearson.

Larsen, D. L., Attkisson, C. C., Hargreaves, W. A. et al. (1979). Assessment of client/patient satisfaction: development of a general scale. *Evaluation and Program Planning*, 2(3).

Lee, W. -I., Shih, B.-Y. & Chung, Y.-S. (2008). The exploration of consumers' behavior in choosing hospital by the application of neural network. *Expert Systems with Applications*, 34(2).

Li, H., Wang, J., Liu, S. et al. (2016). Research and influential factors of health care seeking intention of outpatient among community health service institutions in Harbin. *Chinese Journal of Public Health Management*, 32(6).

Li, J., Li, Z., Qiao, H. et al. (2016). Outpatient satisfaction study in public county hospital reform pilot hospitals, Ningxia. *Journal of Ningxia*

Medical University, 38(12).

Li, X., Zhang, H., Wang, J. et al. (2014). Assessing patient satisfaction with medication related services in hospital settings: a cross-sectional questionnaire survey in China. *International Journal of Clinical Pharmacology and Therapeutics*, 52(7).

Li, Y., Miao, Y., Yang, F. et al. (2015). Progress on the research of health-seeking behaviors of rural patients' with chronic diseases and its influencing factors. *The Chinese Health Service Management*, 8.

Likert, R. (1932). A technique for the measurement of attitudes. *Archives of psychology*, 140.

Linder-Pelz, S. (1982). Toward a theory of patient satisfaction. *Social Science & Medicine*, 16(5).

Liu, Q., Wang, B., Kong, Y. et al. (2011). China's primary health-care reform. *The Lancet*, 377(9783).

Locke, E. A. (1969). What is job satisfaction? *Organizational Behavior and Human Performance*, 4(4).

Lv, Y., Xue, C., Ge, Y. et al. (2016). Analysis of factors influencing inpatient and outpatient satisfaction with the Chinese military health service. *PLOS ONE*, 11(3).

Mansour, M. (2015). Factor analysis of nursing students' perception of patient safety education. *Nurse Education Today*, 35(1).

Meng, Q., Xu, L., Zhang, Y. et al. (2012). Trends in access to health services and financial protection in China between 2003 and 2011: a cross-sectional study. *The Lancet*, 379(9818).

Merks, P., Kazmierczak, J., Olszewska, A. E. et al. (2014). Comparison of factors influencing patient choice of community pharmacy in Poland and in the UK, and identification of components of pharmaceutical care. *Patient Preference and Adherence*, 8.

Meterko, M., Nelson, E. C., Rubin, H. R. et al. (1990). Patient judgments of hospital quality: report of a pilot study. *Medical Care*, 28(9).

Middleton, B., Bloomrosen, M., Dente, M. A. et al. (2013). Enhancing patient safety and quality of care by improving the usability of electronic health record systems: recommendations from AMIA. *Journal of the American Medical Informatics Association*, 20(e1).

Mohd, A. & Chakravarty, A. (2014). Patient satisfaction with services of the outpatient department. *Medical Journal, Armed Forces India*, 70(3).

Mwabu, G., Ainsworth, M. & Nyamete, A. (1993). Quality of medical care and choice of medical treatment in Kenya: an empirical analysis. *Journal of Human Resources*, 28.

Nie, L., Wu, H., Wang, Y. et al. (2018). Analyzing the satisfaction on health management for rural patients with chronic diseases and its influencing factors. *The Chinese Health Service Management*, 3.

Oberoi, S., Chaudhary, N., Patnaik, S. et al. (2016). Understanding health seeking behavior. *Journal of Family Medicine and Primary Care*, 5(2).

Oliver, R. L. (1981). Measurement and evaluation of satisfaction processes in retail settings. *Journal of Retailing*, 57(3).

Pallant, J. (2013). *SPSS survival manual*. London: McGraw-Hill Education.

Pascoe, G. C. (1983). Patient satisfaction in primary health care: a literature review and analysis. *Evaluation and Program Planning*, 6(3-4).

Peng, Q. (2012). Health status and community health services utilization of Nanhai rural residents. Hunan Normal University.

Pillai, R. K., Williams, S. V., Glick, H. A. et al. (2003). Factors affecting decisions to seek treatment for sick children in Kerala, India. *Social Science & Medicine*, 57(5).

Poortaghi, S., Raiesifar, A., Bozorgzad, P. et al. (2015). Evolutionary concept analysis of health seeking behavior in nursing: a systematic review. *BMC Health Services Research*, 15(1).

Prochaska, J. O. & Norcross, J. C. (2018). *Systems of psychotherapy: a transtheoretical analysis*. New York: Oxford University Press.

Qian, D., Pong, R. W., Yin, A. et al. (2009). Determinants of health care demand in poor, rural China: the case of Gansu Province. *Health Policy and Planning*, 24(5).

Qingyue, M. & Shenglan, T. (2013). Universal health care coverage in China: challenges and opportunities. *Procedia—Social and Behavioral Sciences*, 77.

Rahmqvist, M. & Bara, A. -C. (2010). Patient characteristics and quality dimensions related to patient satisfaction. *International Journal for Quality in*

Health Care, January, 86-92.

Schiffman, L. G. & Wisenblit, J. L. (2018). *Consumer Behavior*. London: Pearson.

Shaikh, B. T. & Hatcher, J. (2004). Health seeking behaviour and health service utilization in Pakistan: challenging the policy makers. *Journal of Public Health*, 27(1).

Shi, J., Gong, Y., Li, Y. et al. (2015). Development of out patient satisfaction assessment scale and empirical study. *The Chinese Health Service Management*, 4.

Solomon, M. R., Dahl, D. W., White, K. et al. (2014). *Consumer behavior: buying, having, and being* (Vol. 10). London: Pearson.

Stanworth, J. O., Hsu, R. S. & Warden, C. A. (2017). Validation of a measure of Chinese outpatients'satisfaction in the Taiwan setting. *Inquiry*, 54.

Strasser, S., Aharony, L. & Greenberger, D. (1993). The patient satisfaction process: moving toward a comprehensive model. *Medical Care Review*, 50(2).

Sun, J., Hu, G., Ma, J. et al. (2017). Consumer satisfaction with tertiary healthcare in China: findings from the 2015 China National Patient Survey. *International Journal for Quality in Health Care*, 29(2).

Sun, M. & Han, H. (2013). Healthcare provider choice of Chinese rural residents—empirical study from Gansu, Henan and Guangdong province. *Economic Review*, 2.

Sun, Y., Gregersen, H. & Yuan, W. (2017). Chinese health care system and clinical epidemiology. *Clinical Epidemiology*, 9.

Swan, J. E., Sawyer, J. C., Van Matre, J. G. et al. (1985). Deepening the understanding of hospital patient satisfaction: fulfillment and equity effects. *Journal of Health Care Marketing*, 5(3).

Tehrani, A. B., Feldman, S. R., Camacho, F. T. et al. (2011). Patient satisfaction with outpatient medical care in the United States. *Health Outcomes Research in Medicine*, 2(4).

Thomas, F. (2010). Transnational health and treatment networks: meaning, value and place in health seeking amongst southern African migrants in London. *Health & Place*, 16(3).

Thuan, N. T. B., Lofgren, C., Lindholm, L. et al. (2008). Choice of healthcare provider following reform in Vietnam. *BMC Health Services Research*, 8(1).

Tian, M., Feng, D., Chen, X. et al. (2013). China's rural public health system performance: a cross-sectional study. *PLOS ONE*, 8(12).

Victoor, A., Delnoij, D. M. J., Friele, R. D. et al. (2012). Determinants of patient choice of healthcare providers: a scoping review. *BMC Health Services Research*, 12(1).

Wang, D., Wu, J., Shi, G. et al. (2014). Survey on medical care behavior of the population with flu-like symptoms in Hefei City, Anhui Province. *Chinese Journal of Disease Control & Prevention*, 11.

Wang, Q., Zhang, D. & Hou, Z. (2016). Insurance coverage and socioeconomic differences in patient choice between private and public health care providers in China. *Social Science & Medicine*, 170.

Ware Jr, J. E. & Snyder, M. K. (1975). Dimensions of patient attitudes regarding doctors and medical care services. *Medical Care*, 13(8).

Ware Jr, J. E., Snyder, M. K., Wright, W. R. et al. (1983). Defining and measuring patient satisfaction with medical care. *Evaluation and Program Planning*, 6(3-4).

Wei, J., Shen, L., Yang, H. B. et al. (2015). Development and validation of a Chinese outpatient satisfaction questionnaire: evidence from 46 public general hospitals and 5151 outpatients. *Public Health*, 129(11).

Westbrook, R. A. (1980). Intrapersonal affective influences on consumer satisfaction with products. *Journal of Consumer Research*, 7(1).

Woldeyohanes, T. R., Woldehaimanot, T. E., Kerie, M. W. et al. (2015). Perceived patient satisfaction with in-patient services at Jimma University Specialized Hospital, Southwest Ethiopia. *BMC Research Notes*, 8(1).

Wong, E.L., Leung, M. C., Cheung, A. W. et al. (2011). A population-based survey using PPE-15: relationship of care aspects to patient satisfaction in Hong Kong. *International Journal for Quality in Health Care*, 23(4).

Woodruff, R. B., Cadotte, E. R. & Jenkins, R. L. (1983). Modeling consumer satisfaction processes using experience-based norms. *Journal of Marketing Research*, 20(3).

World Bank Group. (2017). World development indicators 2017.

World Health Organization. (2015). *People's Republic of China health system review*: Manila: WHO Regional Office for the Western Pacific.

Wu, M. (2010). *SPSS operation and application: the practice of quantitative analysis of questionnaire data*. Chongqing: Chongqing University Press.

Xie, Z. & Or, C. (2017). Associations between waiting times, service times, and patient satisfaction in an endocrinology outpatient department: a time study and questionnaire survey. *Inquiry*, 54.

Xin, Y., Li, Y., Xie, X. et al. (2016). Research on influential factors of public's health care choice in the community medical institutions. *Chinese Health Service Management*, 2.

Yi, Y. (1990). A critical review of consumer satisfaction. *Review of Marketing*, 4(1).

Yip, W. & Hsiao, W. (2009). China's health care reform: a tentative assessment. *China Economic Review*, 20(4).

Yip, W. & Hsiao, W. C. (2015). What drove the cycles of Chinese health system reforms? *Health Systems & Reform*, 1(1).

Yu, H. (2015). Universal health insurance coverage for 1. 3 billion people: what accounts for China's success? *Health Policy*, 119(9).

Yu, W., Li, M., Xue, C. et al. (2016). Determinants and influencing mechanism of outpatient satisfaction: a survey on tertiary hospitals in the People's Republic of China. *Patient Preference and Adherence*, 10.

Yuan, Y. & Li, L. (2015). Investigation and analysis of outpatient satisfaction in a general hospital in Hunan province. *China Health Industry*, 26.

Zeithaml, V. A. (1988). Consumer perceptions of price, quality, and value: a means-end model and synthesis of evidence. *The Journal of Marketing*, 52(3).

Zhang, D. (2003). Medical service requirements of villager in Qingdao and its influencing factors. *Chinese Journal of Public Health*, 19(5).

Zhang, G. & Zou, W. (2014). Family splitting behavior, family structure and rural middle-aged and elderly's medical behavior: based on the survey in Handan, Hebei province. *Chinese Journal of Population Science*, 5.

Zhang, L. (2013). Analysis of migrant workers' choice of health institutions and its influencing factors: based on the survey in Nanjing. *Journal of University Electronic Science and Technology of China*, 15(1).

Zhang, N., Sun, D. & Zhou, H. (2011). Influencing factors of outpatients' satisfaction rate in large general hospitals. *Chinese Hospitals*, 15(10).

Zhang, W., Hao, Y., Wu, Q. et al. (2014). Reasons and countermeasures of the nervous doctor-patient relationship in China. *Medicine and Society*, 27(4).

Zhao, X., Lang, Y. & Ma, C. (2015). Self-reported morbidity and service utilization among migrant population in Beijing. *Capital Journal of Public Health*, 3.

Zhong, H. (2011). Effect of patient reimbursement method on health-care utilization: evidence from China. *Health Economics*, 20(11).

Zhou, Z., Mei, C., Zhang, Y. et al. (2011). Study on satisfaction degree of outpatients in a top-notched hospital. *Modern Preventive Medicine*, 38(7).

Zhou, Z., Zhu, L., Zhou, Z. et al. (2014). The effects of China's urban basic medical insurance schemes on the equity of health service utilisation: evidence from Shaanxi Province. *International Journal for Equity in Health*, 13(1).

Appendices

Appendix Ⅰ　Questionnaire of the outpatient perception Survey

序号	问题及选项	回答
	患者一般情况	
1	性别：(1)男　　　(2)女	
2	年龄：＿＿岁	
3	文化程度： (1)没上过学　(2)小学　(3)初中　(4)高中/技校 (5)中专/中技　(6)大专　(7)大学及以上	
4	您的职业： (1)务农　(2)务工　(3)经商　(4)服务　(5)教师　(6)学生 (7)企业　(8)机关事业单位　(9)无业　(10)其他＿＿＿＿＿ (11)退休	
5	您参加了哪种医疗保险： (1)公费医疗　(2)城镇职工基本医疗保险　(3)城镇居民基本医疗保险　(4)新型农村合作医疗保险　(5)城乡居民基本医疗保险(特指) (6)商业保险　(7)其他＿＿＿＿＿　(8)没参加	
6	您的月平均收入为： (1)无收入来源　(2)2000元及以下　(3)2001～4000元　(4)4001元及以上	
7	您是否患有经医生诊断的慢性疾病？　　(1)是　　(2)否	

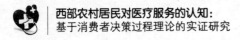
续表

序号	问题及选项	回答
	患者的一般情况	
	常见病就医选择情况	
8	您在患常见病时(病情较轻)一般选择去哪里就诊? (1)村卫生室　　　　(2)乡镇卫生院　　　　(3)县级及以上级别医院	
9	选择原因(可多选): (1)距离近/方便　(2)收费合理　(3)技术水平高　(4)设备条件好 (5)药品丰富　　(6)服务态度好　(7)定点单位　(8)有熟人 (9)有自己信赖的医生　(10)其他_____	
	门诊服务满意度情况	
10	您感觉去就诊路上所花的时间长短如何? (1)很长　(2)较长　(3)一般　(4)较短　(5)很短	
11	您感觉在医院候诊所花的时间长短如何? (1)很长　(2)较长　(3)一般　(4)较短　(5)很短	
12	您认为医护人员向你解释病情等问题时表达清晰吗? (1)很差或没有　(2)差　(3)一般　(4)好　(5)很好	
13	您认为医生给您的治疗方案方面的意见如何? (1)很差或没有　(2)差　(3)一般　(4)好　(5)很好	
14	您认为医务人员的服务态度如何? (1)很差　(2)差　(3)一般　(4)好　(5)很好	
15	您觉得就诊单位的设备条件如何? (1)很差　(2)差　(3)一般　(4)好　(5)很好	
16	您觉得就诊单位的环境(包括厕所)如何? (1)很差　(2)差　(3)一般　(4)好　(5)很好	
17	在接受服务的过程中,您认为您所支付的医疗或药品费用如何? (1)很贵　(2)贵　(3)一般　(4)较便宜　(5)很便宜	
18	在接受服务的过程中,您认为医务人员的技术水平如何? (1)很差　(2)差　(3)一般　(4)好　(5)很好	

Appendix Ⅱ   Patient informed consent

知情同意书

尊敬的患者/家属：

您好！本次调查的目的是了解目前门诊患者对医疗卫生服务的选择与满意情况，探讨医疗护理质量与患者需求的关系，以便为提高农村地区卫生服务的质量与效率，制定相关政策、完善管理制度提供必要的依据。本问卷为匿名问卷，请如实填写相关信息，选出您在患常见病时的就医机构，并对门诊服务进行满意度评分。根据《中华人民共和国统计法》的有关规定，本次调查将信守保密原则，所取得的数据仅用于统计分析，研究结果将进行学术汇报或发表，您填写的内容将不会以任何形式向政府、其他机构及个人透露。

非常感谢您回答这份问卷，谢谢合作！

机构地址：_____省（自治区）_____市_____县

机构全称（《医疗机构执业许可证》上登记的名称）：_____

组织机构代码：□□□□□□□□-□

机构类别：□县医院　　□中医院　　□妇幼保健院

调查员（签名）：_____　　填表日期：2014 年_____月_____日

监督员（签名）：_____　　填表日期：2014 年_____月_____日

Part II Inpatients Study

List of Abbreviations

CGH	County-level general hospital
CMCCH	County-level maternal and child care hospital
CMS	Cooperative medical scheme
CSQ	Client satisfaction questionnaire
CTCMH	County-level traditional Chinese medicine hospital
EFA	Exploratory factor analysis
FMC	Free medical care
HCAHPS	Hospital consumer assessment of health care providers and systems
HCF	Health care facility
HCSB	Health care seeking behavior
GDP	Gross domestic product
NCMS	New cooperative medical scheme
NEMS	National essential medicines system
NHC	National Health Commission of the People's Republic of China
NHSS	National health service survey
OOP	Out-of-pocket
PHC	Primary health care
PJHQ	Patient judgment of hospital quality
TH	Township hospital
UEBMI	Urban employee basic medical insurance
URBMI	Urban resident basic medical insurance

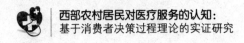

VSSS   Verona service satisfaction scale

WHO   World Health Organization

Chapter 1 Introduction

1.1 Background

1.1.1 Health care reform in China

Uneven distributions of health care resources and insufficient capacities of health care services have been a long-standing problem in China. The problem began from the commercialisation of the health system in the late 1970s.

In 1978, China started the economic reform towards a market-oriented economy. Since then, China's economic development has been remarkable. Until 2013, unprecedented growth occurred, with the gross domestic product (GDP) increasing by around 9.5% to 11.5% every year. China's rapid economic growth has brought substantial improvements in living standards for the Chinese people. In some respects, the economic growth acted as a positive stimulus to the Chinese health sector, because increasing per capita income meant more potential resources per capita for health. (Wagstaff, Lindelow, Wang & Zhang, 2009)

However, at the same time, the economic reforms brought challenges to health service system. The rapid shift away from collective agriculture resulted in an almost complete collapse of the cooperative medical scheme, which was the mainstay of free health care for the rural population. Shifts in the tax base as a result of the economic transition and weak tax collection incentives for the local government led to a steady decline in government revenues as a share of GDP. Therefore, the government reduced the budget of social sectors, including health care sectors. This led to the policy of "financial autonomy" for health care facilities, which were allowed to supplement their budget allocations by charging patients for the medicines and the services that they provided; and the "price schedule", on which health care providers could make profits from drugs and high-tech care. (Wagstaff et al., 2009) These led to perverse incentives for doctors to over-treat, resulting in escalating costs and medical poverty. (Huang, 2011) Between 1978 and 2003, out-of-pocket (OOP) expenditures grew in real terms at an annual rate of 15.7%. (Wagstaff et al., 2009) By 2003, 30% of poor households in the government's National Health Service Survey (NHSS) thought that health care costs was the main cause of their poverty. (Huang, 2011) Especially in rural areas, health care costs was unaffordable for many households, thus increasing poverty and sharpening rural inequalities. Consequently, increasing health care costs topped the list of public concerns in government surveys.

In addition, beginning with the economic reform, the primary health care system in China was dismantled in both urban and rural areas. (Wagstaff et al., 2009) Lack of confidence in PHC led to the deterioration of these facilities. As a result, patients with minor diseases invaded secondary and tertiary hospitals. (Hesketh & Zhu, 1997) The medical burden and difficultly in seeking medical care became more and more serious. mean parallel concerns began to surface in health care field, such as inequalities between the richer eastern and the poorer western provinces, growing rural-urban disparities, and so on. Widespread discontent led to the recognition that a reform was imperative.

The new health care reform plans had been in place by the end of 2007, and 850 billion *yuan* were allocated from central government for the first three-year phase from 2009 to 2011. (Cheng, 2008) The five core components of the reform were: (1) expanding insurance coverage with a target of achieving universal coverage with significant demand subsidies for the rural population to enroll in the New Cooperative Medical Scheme (NCMS) and for the urban uninsured to enroll in the Urban Resident Basic Medical Insurance Scheme (URBMI); (2) increasing government spending on public health services, especially in lower-income regions, with the goal of equalizing public health spending across regions; (3) establishing PHC facilities—community health centers in urban areas and township health centers in rural areas—which would serve as gate-keepers in the long run; (4) reforming the pharmaceutical market and establishing the national essential medicines system (NEMS); and (5) pilot testing public hospital reforms. (Anonymous, 2009) The major focus of the first phase was strengthening PHC system and increasing health insurance coverage and benefits, so as to provide more equitable access to health care services, and reduce the severe gap between rural and urban health care quality. (Zhou, Li & Hesketh, 2014) And to guide resident HCSB, the social health insurance introduced a differential reimbursement policy tailored to the level of HCFs, which ruled that the higher the facility level the less the insurance reimbursement rates.

With the 2009 health care reform, accessibility and affordability of health care services had been substantially improved through increased government investments, universal health insurance coverage, the basic public service program, and an essential drug system. However, challenges remained. Progress in health care service delivery reform had been slow. Despite substantial investments in infrastructure and training at the PHC level, visits and admissions continued to take place mainly at secondary and tertiary hospitals. PHC facilities had not been able to perform a gate-keeping function, and health care delivery remained hospital-centered and fragmented. As Figure 1-1 shows, for inpatient care services, in 2003, 28.8% of the rural population chose township hospitals (THs), 42.6% chose county-level HCFs, and 14.1% chose municipal or provincial hospitals; in 2008, 36.6% of the rural population chose THCs, 50.0% chose county-level HCFs, and 10.6% chose municipal or provincial hospitals; however, in 2013, 29.8% chose THCs, 55.7% chose county-level HCFs, and 12.9% chose municipal or provincial hospitals.

To solve the problems, in 2012, the 18th NPC & CPPCC emphasized the goal of promoting the comprehensive reform of the health care system, with the focus on the rural area, and required improving the rational allocation of medical resources, and establishing a hierarchical health care service system.

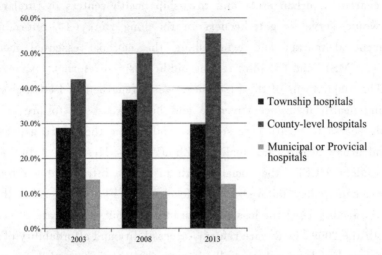

Figure 1-1   Inpatient HCSB in rural areas in 2003, 2008 and 2013

1.1.2   Hierarchy health care system in China

For a long time, China's health care system had always adhered to the construction of the three-level medical service network in urban and rural areas. While under the proposed hierarchy health care system, the various levels of the health care system would be integrated and coordinated, through the overall planning of the urban and rural health care resources, clearly defining the responsibilities of all HCFs, effectively guiding patient health care utilization, and standardizing medical activities, so as to continue improving the fairness and accessibility of health care services.

In urban areas, tertiary hospitals would mainly provide emergency and critical care services for complex diseases; secondary hospitals mainly accept patients referred by the tertiary hospitals, who are during the recovery period of acute diseases, after the operation, or in the convalescence period of critical diseases.

In rural areas, county-level HCFs mainly provide diagnosis and treatment services for patients with common and frequently occurring diseases, emergency care for patients with critical diseases, and referral service for patients with complex diseases.

Moreover, PHC facilities in both urban and rural areas provide diagnosis and treatment services for patients with common and frequently occurring diseases. And they also cooperate with rehabilitation hospitals and nursing homes to provide treatment, rehabilitation and nursing services for patients with the chronic disease, cancer, or rehabilitation.

And the principle for the hierarchical health care system in China can be concluded as first visit at PHC facilities, two-way referral, acute and chronic diseases treated separately, and up and down linkage.

First visit at PHC facilities means through policy guidance, encouraging patients with common and frequently occurring diseases firstly go to PHC facilities for diagnosis and treatment. Two-way referral means through improving referral procedures, focusing on downward referral for patients during the chronic period or recovery period, gradually achieving the orderly transfer among different levels and categories of medical institutions. Acute and chronic diseases treated separately means by improving the service system for sub-acute and chronic diseases, and implementing the function and responsibility of all the HCFs at different levels, patients survived the acute period would be transferred out of the tertiary hospital. The up and down linkage is establishing a division and coordination mechanism among all the HCFs, so as to promote the vertical communication of high-quality health care resources.

In conclusion, the hierarchy health care system in China is designed to reduce inefficiencies in the provision of health care services thus lowing costs; provide timely access service to satisfy patient needs; and to guide patients choosing the right services.

However, different from the gatekeeper system in some western countries, patients are encouraged instead of restricted to see general practitioners in lower-level HCFs. patients are allowed to visit HCFs of any grade.

Therefore, even under the hierarchy health care system, many other factors may affect patient health care seeking behavior.

1.1.3　Health care seeking behavior

Health care seeking behavior (HCSB), defined as health care service utilization, involving the interpersonal interaction with the selected HCF. It is influenced by many factors, such as patient age, gender, education level, occupation, insurance, health status, preference, price and quality of health care service, distance to HCF, commute mode, waiting time and so on. And depending on these factors and their interactions, HCSB is a complex outcome of many factors operating at individual, family, and community levels. (Siddiqui, Sohag & Siddiqui, 2011)

As one of the important factors determining the acceptance and outcome of health care services, HCSB is also an important and commonly used indicator to evaluate patient health care demands, health care quality and health care resource allocations. (Nguma, 2010) Appropriate HCSB could reduce delays in diagnosis, improve treatment compliance, benefit health promotion strategies, and consequently promote the equity and efficiency of health care delivery.

As previously mentioned, beginning with the economic reforms in 1978, the PHC system in China was dismantled in both urban and rural areas. Lack of confidence in PHC system led to the deterioration of these facilities, as a result, patients with even minor conditions swamped secondary and tertiary hospitals. Even after the new health care reform, patient visits and admissions continued to take place mainly at secondary and tertiary hospitals. PHC facilities had not been able to perform a gate-keeping function, and health care delivery remained hospital-centered and fragmented. Therefore, except for improving the structure of health care system, understanding patient HCSB and their influencing factors are also of great importance.

1.1.4 Previous studies on patient HCSB

Studies on patient HCSB and the relevant influential factors are abundant both at home and abroad. It is found that the influential factors could be divided into two categories: individual characteristics and health care system related factors. Individual characteristics include patient age, gender, educational level, income level, type and severity of diseases, health insurance, medical payment method, and so on. The second category includes price and the quality of health care service, distance to HCF, commute mode, waiting time, and so on.

However, most of the studies in China focused on the outpatient HCSB, and attempted to analyze patient HCSB and relevant influential factors in urban areas.

1.1.4.1 Studies on individual influential factors of patient HCSB

Among the individual characteristics, age, gender, education level, income level, type and severity of disease are social-demographic factors, which have been the spotlight of many studies both at home and abroad. (Bao et al., 2010; Brown & Theoharides, 2010; Ellis, Mcinnes & Stephenson, 2010; Habtom & Ruys, 2007; Mehra, Bhatnagar, Rao & Garg, 2016; Pourreza, Khabiri, Arab & Sari, 2009; Roudriguez & Stoyanova, 2004; Rous & Hotchkiss, 2010; Singh & Ladusingh, 2009; Zhao, Chen & Liu, 2009) However, the results of these studies were not consistent.

Pourreza et al. (2009) found that age, sex, perceived severity of illness, income, educational level, household size and payment method were the most statistically significant variables affecting Iranian residents' seeking care from health care centers. Habtom and Ruys (2007) revealed that education, perceived quality, distance, user fees, severity of illness, socio-economic status and place of residence were statistically significant in the choice of a health care provider. Rodriguez and Stoyanova (2004) found that age, sex, and health and public supply characteristics had a distinct impact on patient utilization of physician services in Spain. Brown and Theoharides (2010) carried out a household survey in 25 counties in China, and the results showed that age, the share of household expenditures allocated to food consumption, and the presence of other sick people in the household negatively affected the decision to seek health care while the disability had a positive influence. Ellis et al. (2010) confirmed that age, sex, education could strongly influence the health care utilization of residents in Cairo. Zhao et al. (2009) found that gender, age, and payment method were associated with resident HCSB in Jinan; women preferred the community health centers, and men preferred the comprehensive hospitals; patients below 20 preferred the community health centers, patients between 20 and 60 preferred the comprehensive hospitals, and patients above 60 preferred self-medication. While Bao et al. (2010) found that age, education level, and marital status had significant effects on patient HCSB in Shanghai; the patients below 35 would like to choose the tertiary hospitals, and those above 35 would like to visit the community health centers; the patients with the high school degree or below preferred the community health centers, and those with the college degree or above preferred the tertiary hospitals; unmarried patients preferred the tertiary hospitals, and the others preferred the community health centers.

Furthermore, health insurance, as an important factor affecting resident HCSB, has always drawn plenty of attentions. Both domestic and foreign studies have found that the resident HCSB were sensitive to the health insurance policy. (Brown & Theoharides, 2010; Deolalikar & Martinsson, 2004; Ellis et al., 2010; Jowett, Lai & Chen, 2010; Mitchell & Hadley, 1997; Rodriguez & Stoyanova, 2004; Shan, 2009; Zhou & Yan, 2008).

Jowett et al. (2004) revealed that the insured patients were more likely to use outpatient health care services in Vietnam. Mitchell and Hadley (1997) compared the effects of different health care insurances on the HCSB of young females suffering from breast cancer in the US, and the result showed that female enrolled in the HMO insurance would like to visit the HCF within a short distance rather than the one far away but with a high grade. Rodriguez and Stoyanova (2004) found that the patients with only public insurance went to the general practitioner 2.8 times more than the specialist; individuals with duplicate coverage had a ratio of general practitioner/specialist visits equal to 1.4; and those with only private health insurance contacted specialists more often than general practitioners. Moreover, insurance reimbursement ratio and medial payment method had significant effects on patient HCSB. Shan (2009) found that the community health centers were the first choice for 51.36% of the participants in Shenzhen due to the low price and convenient medical treatment process, and for those covered by a health insurance, the proportion choosing the community health center was even higher. Brown and Theoharides (2010) found that the health insurance reimbursement scheme and average daily medical expenditure strongly influenced resident hospital choice. And Ellis et al. (2010) also found health insurance was strongly associated with the health care utilization of residents in Cairo.

But there were also domestic studies pointing out that inpatients were less sensitive to medical insurance, especially in developed provinces. (Lai & Chen, 2010; Wang et al., 2018; Zhou & Yan, 2008). Zhou and Yan (2008) found that there was no difference for patients with different types of health insurances to choose inpatient care services or not. Lai and Chen (2010) revealed that for rural residents in Panyu, Guangzhou, the health insurance reimbursement scheme did not affect their choice of HCFs too much. Wang et al. (2018) disclosed that the social health insurance had no statistically significant effect on the inpatient health care utilization among the internal migrants.

1.1.4.2　Studies on health care system related influential factors of patient HCSB

Factors related to health care service system, including the price of health care, the quality of health care, and the distance to HCF were verified to be of great importance for patient HCSB.

Lavy and Quigley (1991) disclosed that the price of health care service had an impact on the choice and frequency of patient health care, especially for the outpatients. However, for the inpatient choice of health care, the impact of the price of health care service decreased obviously. Ellis et al. (2010) found that the outpatients in Cairo were very sensitive to the price of health care service, while the inpatients did not show evident price sensitivity. And Sahn, Younger and Genicot (2010) found that in rural Tanzania, the patients with lower income were more sensitive to health care service price.

Besides the price, the quality of health care also had significant effects on patient HCSB. Hanson, Yip and Hsiao (2004) showed that the outpatient health care demand was significantly associated with the cost performance of HCFs. Ellis et al. (2010) disclosed that in Cairo patients with high income preferred HCFs with high qualities.

Moreover, many studies pointed out that the accessibility to HCFs was important for patient choice of health care services. (Nonvignon et al., 2010; Mehra et al., 2016; Sarma, 2003)

Sarma (2003) investigated factors affecting the outpatient health care demands of rural Indians, and the result showed that the income and health care price were two statistically significant determinants of health care choice, and the distance to HCFs was a pronounced inhibiting factor for the demand of health care. Nonvignon et al. (2010) explored the HCSB of patients under 5 years old in rural Ghana, and the result presented that longer travel, waiting and treatment time prohibited the patients from choosing health care services.

In China, only a few studies were quantitative researches on the association between patient HCSB and the price, quality, and accessibility of health care service. Most studies focused on the subjective perception of the price, quality, and accessibility of health care service. (Bao & Tao, 2009; Bao, 2010; Jia, 2010; Lai & Chen, 2010; Liu, Yang & Zhang, 2011; Zhang, 2005; Zhao et al., 2009)

For example, the study carried out in Ping County, Jiangxi showed that the professional skill, accessibility, and medical equipments of HCF were the major factors affecting rural resident HCSB. (Jia, 2010) Zhang (2005) found that in rural central China the professional skill level of HCF was of significant importance for patient HCSB; the patients with severe disease tended to choose comprehensive hospitals with high professional skill levels. Lai and Chen (2010) found that the rural resident HCSB was affected by both individual characteristic (income, disease severity, and personal perception of health care) and health care system related factors (accessibility, quality of HCFs). Liu et al. (2011) found that in Shenyang the most important factor affecting urban residents was the accessibility of an HCF.

1.1.5 Patient satisfaction

As patient-centered care has gained more and more emphasis from policy makers, clinicians, and researchers, besides patient health care seeking behavior, patient satisfaction has been recognized as one of the key element of health care quality. (Alabri & Albalushi, 2014; Bleich, ÖZaltin & Murray, 2009; Co et al., 2003; Greco et al., 2015; Haj, Bahri, Rais & Lamrini, 2013; Harrison et al., 2009; Paddison et al., 2015; Pozzi, 2015; Shipley et al., 2000; Stang et al., 2016; Williams & Wilkinson, 1995; Yeddula, 2012). From 2003, evaluation on patient satisfaction has been recruited in the NHSS.

Patient satisfaction is the level of contentment that patients feel about the health care services received from their health care providers. It is a comprehensive evaluation of health care experiences, including treatment process, health care cost, health care outcome, service attitude and so on. It represents whether the delivered health care services meet the subjective and objective needs, expectations and requirements of a patient. (Haj et al., 2013)

Also, patient satisfaction, as a multidimensional concept, is influenced by many factors, such as patient characteristics (age, gender, education level, etc.), quality of health care services (convenience, accessibility, affordability, etc.), and so on.

As a powerful tool to evaluate the quality of health care and the work performance of medical staff, patient satisfaction assessment is widely used both at home and abroad. With patient satisfaction evaluation, HCFs could understand the needs and requirements of patients, and find the shortage of their health care services, so as to improve the quality of health care services. Moreover, patient satisfaction evaluation can strengthen the communication between HCFs and patients, resolve the contradiction between doctors and patients, and establish a harmonious doctor-patient relationship.

However, evaluation of patient satisfaction is very different from the satisfaction evaluation in the other general service fields. Firstly, the asymmetry of health care service information due to the professional and technical nature of health care services might lead to higher expectations of patients and comparatively lower patient satisfaction. Secondly, for patients, the health care outcomes are the most important; that is to say, without consideration of all the influencing factors, the treatment effects may directly affect or even determine patient satisfaction. In the end, due to the dominant status of HCFs, especially the public hospitals, patients may not be able to evaluate satisfaction according to their actual feeling. Therefore, the authenticity of the patient satisfaction assessment needs to be further screened.

1.1.6 Previous studies on patient satisfaction

A large number of empirical studies on patient satisfaction have been carried out at home and abroad, and the results showed that major factors affecting patient satisfaction included individual factors (age, gender, race, education, income, self-perception of physical or psychological health status, type and severity of disease, and previous experience in receiving health care, health insurance, etc.), and health care system related factors (HCF environment, waiting time, medical equipment, professional skill and service attitude of medical staff, doctor-patient relationship, health care expense, treatment outcome, and reputation, location, and grade of HCF, etc.).

1.1.6.1　Studies on individual influential factors of patient satisfaction

Many studies have found that age is a significant factor that affects patient satisfaction. Elder patients tended to have higher satisfaction, because they might have lower expectations for health care services, or they would not express their dissatisfaction. (Larsson, Larsson & Starrin, 1995; Nguyen Thi, Briancon, Empereur & Guillemin, 2002; Pope & Russell, 1997; Rahmqvist, 2001; Wilde, Owens & Batchelor, 1996; Williams & Calnan, 1991)

And some studies also found that patient health status was significantly associated with their satisfaction with health care services. (Cleary et al., 1992; Hall, Milburn & Epstein, 1993; Linderpelz, 1982; Zapka et al., 1995)

Hall et al. (1993) showed that a patient health status was an important factor that determined the patient satisfaction, which meant that patients with better health status would be more satisfied with their health care services. Zapka et al. (1995) disclosed that the patient with a comparatively good health status usually had high satisfaction, so did the patient with chronic diseases. Linderpelz (1982) pointed out that patient expectations for health would affect their satisfaction. And Cleary et al. (1992) found that patients suffering from AIDS usually had lower satisfaction when they had severe disease status or psychological pressure.

However, some studies found that compared with the physical health status of patients, their psychological status had more significant impacts on patient satisfaction. (Cohen, Forbes & Garraway, 1996; Greenberg & Rosenheck, 2004; Marshall, Hays & Mazel, 1996; Nguyen Thi et al., 2002)

Greenberg and Rosenheck (2004) and Nguyen Thi et al. (2002) found that the patient health status especially the psychological status was significantly associated with his/her satisfaction. However, Cohen et al. (1996) found that patient satisfaction had a fairly low association with his/her physical health status, but a significantly high association with the psychological status. Likewise, Marshall et al. (1996) also found that patient psychological instead of physical health status would affect his/her satisfaction.

In China, studies on patient satisfaction regarding individual factors mainly focused on age, education level, income level, and so on. (Zhang, 2007; Qiao, Liu & Chen, 2010)

Zhang (2007) revealed that for patients of different age groups, there were significant differences in the satisfaction with environment of HCFs, service attitude, waiting time, treatment procedure, treatment outcome, and overall satisfaction; for patients living in different areas, there were significant differences in the satisfaction with waiting time, treatment procedure, and treatment outcome; and for patients of different admission types, their satisfaction with the environment of HCF and the treatment procedure was significantly different. Wang and Jiang (2010) disclosed that for the rural residents, age, residential area, occupation, and income were salient factors that affected patient satisfaction. Qiao et al. (2010) found that for the urban residents in Beijing, age was positively associated with the patient satisfaction with community health centers, and income was also significantly associated with patient satisfaction. However, Han et al. (2009) found that age was negatively correlated with the inpatient satisfaction; income was positively correlated with the inpatient satisfaction, and patients living in rural areas showed lower satisfaction. And Zhu et al. (2010) found that in urban Nanjing, gender was significantly associated with the patient satisfaction with community health centers. Liao et al. (2010) considered that in the hospital in Shenzhen, education and income levels were main factors that affected outpatient satisfaction. Similarly, Chen and Xue (2009) exhibited the results that for patients visiting community health centers, there were significant differences in the satisfaction of patients with different education and income levels.

Health insurance, as another important factor affecting patient satisfaction, has attracted considerable attention. (Huang, 2009; Li & Jin, 2007; Qiao et al., 2010) Huang (2009) found that for both the inpatients and outpatients, the satisfaction of those without any health insurance was significantly lower than those with a health insurance. Qiao et al. (2010) pointed out that the satisfaction of patients enrolled in different types of health insurance were significantly distinct, with the highest satisfaction for the patients enrolled in the free medical care, and the lowest satisfaction for the patients enrolled in the commercial insurance.

However, some scholars have found that health insurance had no impact on patient satisfaction. Li and Jin (2007) evaluated the inpatient satisfaction with the HCF environment, service quality, service attitude, and medical cost, and the results showed that health insurance could not influence the patient satisfaction.

1.1.6.2　Studies on health care system related influential factors of patient satisfaction

Patient expectation and previous experience in receiving health care were found directly associated with patient satisfaction, which meant that when the patient perception about current health care services was worse than their expectations or previous experience, they would have a low satisfaction. (Crow et al., 2001) But Froehlich and Welch (1996) did not found any correlation between patient expectation and satisfaction.

However, many studies did not recruit patient expectation or previous experience into the analysis, and they only focused on patient perception of satisfaction. (Andaleeb, 1998; Falvo & Smith, 1983; Hasin, Seeluangsawat & Shareef, 2001; Liao et al., 2010; Mummalaneni & Gopalakrishna, 1995; Porter & Beuf, 1994; Zhou, Mei & Zhang, 2011; Zhu et al., 2010)

Andaleeb (1998) built and validated a five-factor patient satisfaction model, which stated doctor-patient communication, medical staff professional skill, medical equipment, enthusiasm of medical staff, and medical expense could affect patient satisfaction. Porter and Beuf (1994) and Mummalaneni and Gopalakrishna (1995) have found that the patient satisfaction was determined by many factors, including HCF environment, medical equipment, medical staff service attitude and communication skill, mode of transportation, and so on. Falvo and Smith (1983) found that doctor-patient interaction was a key factor that influenced patient satisfaction. Hasin et al. (2001) found that health care quality and HCF environment were critical influential factors for patient satisfaction. Zhou et al. (2011) showed that health care expense, HCF environment, medical staff professional skill, and service quality of nurses affected the outpatient satisfaction. Zhu et al. (2010) disclosed that the critical factors affecting the patient satisfaction with the community health centers in urban Nanjing included health insurance deductible, physician professional skill, and type of essential medicines. And Liao et al. (2010) found that in Shenzhen, the outpatient satisfaction was mainly affected by registration fee, physician service attitude, service attitude of pharmacy staff, and HCF environment.

1.2　Research objectives

In this study, we chose to focus on the inpatient health care seeking behavior and satisfaction in rural western China, a region where poverty, ethnic diversity, and geographical access represent particular challenges to ensure universal access to health care. (Gao et al., 2017; Wang et al., 2011)

Western China includes Chongqing, Ningxia Hui Autonomous Region, Guangxi Zhuang Autonomous Region, Xinjiang Weiwuer Autonomous Region, Gansu Province, Shaanxi Province, Sichuan Province, Guizhou Province, Yunnan Province, Qinghai Province, Inner Mongolia and Tibet Autonomous Region. With a vast geographical area and a sparse population, western China contains nearly 42 million rural residents and is populated by Chinese ethnic minority groups. In 2010, the population density in western China was 142 people per kilometer, compared with 300 per kilometer in central China and 581 per kilometer in eastern China; western China had a higher proportion of rural population (58.6%) than central China (54.7%) and eastern China (40.0%); the median proportion of the population belonging to ethnic minority groups was 34.2% in western China, compared with 2.4% in central China and 2.2% in eastern China; and 71.1% of China's ethnic minority population lived in western China, representing 31.1% of the population in the region.

And western China is an underdeveloped area, whose median gross domestic product (GDP) per capita is much lower than those of eastern and central China. In 2010, the GDP per capita in western China was 22,700 *yuan*, compared with 25,100 *yuan* for central China and 44,100 *yuan* for eastern China.

It can be seen from the above that there are significant differences in both the natural and social environment between western China and eastern and central China, which has a great influence on the allocation of health resources.

According to previous studies, the health care service supply system in poor western China lacked sufficient operating funds and service capabilities, and most rural families had low educational levels, leading to poor access to necessary health knowledge and information. (Zhu, 2010) At the same time, western China also faced a shortage of medical workers, and a poorly formulated health care system, and the medical staff's overall level of education and job title were far below that of the national average level. (Chen, 2014)

Thus, it is necessary to perform this study in western China.

Moreover, as stated above, most of the Chinese studies focused on outpatients, and attempted to analyze patient HCSB, satisfaction, and the relevant influential factors in urban areas. Therefore, this study aimed to investigate the inpatient HCSB in rural western China, as well as their satisfaction with the inpatient care services that they received, and furthermore to confirm the factors that affected their utilization and satisfaction, and finally to put forward evidence-based policy recommendations for improvements.

1.3 Research methodology and design

As is shown in Figure 1-2, to achieve the objectives, this study reviewed the literature to illustrate the concepts and relevant policies, as well as to summarize the relevant researches' progress at home and abroad. Then the statistical analyses, including descriptive statistics, univariate and multivariate analysis, exploratory factor analysis (EFA) etc. were conducted with IBM SPSS 21.0 by processing the data from field studies. Evaluations were made afterwards according to the results of theoretical and statistical analyses. And policy implications were also proposed based on the research to deal with the practical issues.

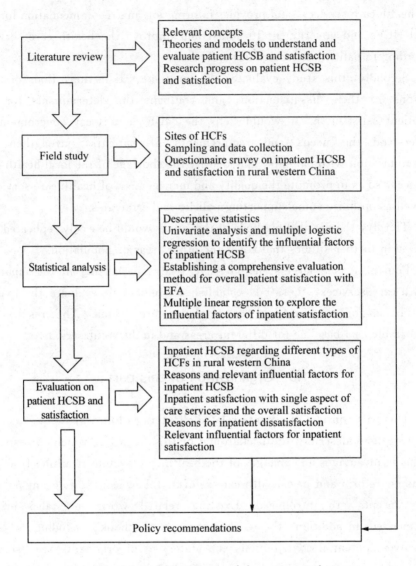

Figure 1-2   Flow diagram of the current study

1.4   Potential contributions

Firstly, the study investigates the inpatient HCSB in rural western China, and identifies the reasons and influential factors for the inpatient to choose the corresponding HCF. It discloses patient preferences and demands for health care services, and provides information and recommendation for the local HCFs and government to adjust and improve the health care services according to patient characteristics and needs.

Secondly, this study evaluates the inpatient satisfaction, finds out the reasons for their dissatisfaction, and confirms the determinants for the inpatient satisfaction. It would help the HCFs and local government to understand the needs and requirements of patients, strengthen the communication with patients, and identify the shortage of the local health care services, so as to promote the quality and management of health care services, as well as optimize some supporting policies and strategies.

Thirdly, the detailed methods of this study would be easily replicated and utilized in further studies that cover the other areas or population.

Fourthly, as a large-scale intensive study specializing in the inpatient health care services, the study establishes a model to evaluate the overall satisfaction for the inpatient in rural western China. The results are comparable as a baseline for different areas and in different periods.

1.5 Organization of this part

This part consists of six interrelated chapters as follows:

Chapter 1 describes the background of this research, which corresponds to the disadvantages and changes of the health care system resulting from the economic reform and new health care reform. Likewise, the relevant policies and concepts are introduced. Existing related works are also briefly summarized. In addition, the whole picture of the book, including research objectives, potential contributions and statement of originality are listed in this section, accompanied with research methodology and book organization.

Chapter 2 provides a literature review, which covers the concepts of patient HCSB and satisfaction, and introduces the theories and models to understand HCSB and satisfaction. On the basis, the detailed methods of this study are established. And the knowledge gaps are also identified in this chapter.

Chapter 3 firstly declares the objectives of this study, and then explains the research methods in detail, and specifies the implementation approach of this research, including data sampling and collection, data processing, statistical analysis and quality assurance.

The study findings are presented in Chapters 4 and 5.

Chapter 4 presents the results regarding the inpatient HCSB and the reasons for the inpatients choosing the corresponding HCFs in rural western China. And the influential factors for the inpatient HCSB are also determined. It provides information and evidence to understand the local patient health needs, demands and preferences.

Chapter 5 presents the inpatient satisfaction with each single aspect of health care services, subdomains and the overall health care services. The relevant influential factors are also investigated. By exploring the overall inpatient satisfaction, a comprehensive evaluation method is established by EFA, generating a synthetic assessment value for further studies.

Chapter 6 generalizes the conclusion and puts forward the policy recommendations. Meanwhile, the limitations of the current study and the perspectives for future work are also illustrated.

Chapter 2　Literature review

A literature review is provided in this chapter. The literature review covers the theories and models to explore patient HCSB and satisfaction, as well as the relevant influential factors. The knowledge gaps are also identified in this chapter.

2.1　Health care seeking behavior

2.1.1　Concept of HCSB

The definition of HCSB is often considered vague and difficult to define. There is no common definition agreed upon by socialists in any sociological literature. Different definitions may be used in different studies.

Some studies have defined HCSB as any remedial actions that individuals undertake to rectify a perceived health problem. (Ward, Mertens & Thomas, 1997)

Oberoi, Chaudhary, Patnaik and Singh (2016) and Olenja (2003) defined HCSB as any action undertaken by individuals who perceived themselves to have a health problem or to be ill for the purpose of finding an appropriate remedy.

Chinn and Kramer (2010) and Poortaghi et al. (2015) defined HCSB as an individual deed to the promotion of maximum well being, recovery, and rehabilitation.

And in some other studies, HCSB referred to utilization of health care system. (Bayu, Fasil & Abrha, 2016; Chomi et al., 2014; Mackian, 2001;

Siddiqui et al., 2011)

In this study, HCSB is defined as utilization of health care services, which involves the interpersonal interaction with the selected HCFs.

2.1.2　Theories and models to understand HCSB

Various theories and models have been developed to help to explain HCSB and suggest strategies to achieve desired behavioral changes. (Poortaghi et al., 2015) Frequently used frameworks include Theory of Reasoned Action (TRA), Theory of Planned Behavior (TPB), Health Belief Model (HBM), and Andersen Behavioral Model (ABM), etc.

2.1.2.1　Theory of Reasoned Action

Theory of Reasoned Action was developed by Martin Fishbein and Icek Ajzen in 1967, which aimed to explain the relationship between attitudes and behaviors within human activity. The TRA is used to predict how individuals will behave based on their pre-existing attitudes and behavioral intentions (see Figure 2-1). According to the TRA, the individual intention to perform a behavior is the main predictor of whether or not the person actually performs the behavior. (Montano & Kasprzyk, 2008) The intention is known as a behavioral intention and comes as a result of a belief that performing the behavior will lead to a specific outcome. The behavioral intention is important to the theory because the intention is determined by the attitude to behaviors and subjective norms. (Lacaille, 2013) The TRA suggests that stronger intentions lead to increased efforts and possibility to perform a behavior.

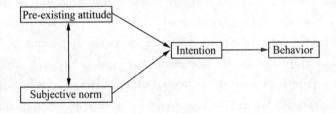

Figure 2-1　Theory of reasoned action

The TRA has been used in many studies as a framework to explore health behaviors, for example, sexual behavior. (Doswell, Braxter, Cha & Kim, 2011), exercise behavior (Bentler & Speckart, 1981), condom use

(Albarracin, Johnson, Fishbein & Muellerleile, 2001), etc. However, the major problem of TRA is the ignorance of the connections between individuals, both the interpersonal and social relations in which they act, and the broader social structures that govern the social practice. Although TRA recognizes the importance of social norms, strategies are limited to a consideration of individual perceptions of these social phenomena. (Terry, Gallois & Mccamish, 1995). Additionally, the habituation of past behavior tends to reduce the impact that an intention has on a behavior as the habit increases. Gradually, the performance of a behavior becomes less of a rational, initiative behavior but more of a learned response. (Bagozzi, 1981)

2.1.2.2 Theory of Planned Behavior

Theory of Planned Behavior, which was proposed by Lcek Ajzen in 1985 to improve the predictive power of the TRA by including perceived behavioral control, emerged as a major framework for understanding, predicting, and changing human social behavior.

As Figure 2-2 shows, the central factor in the theory is the individual intention to perform a given behavior. Intentions are assumed to capture the motivational factors that influence a behavior; they are indications of how dare people are willing to try, and how much of an effort they are planning to exert, in order to perform the behavior. As a general rule, the stronger the intention to engage in a behavior, the more likely the performance would be.

There are three conceptually independent determinants of the intention. The first is the attitude toward a behavior, which refers to the degree to which a person has a favorable or unfavorable evaluation or appraisal of the behavior in question. The second predictor is a social factor termed the subjective norm. It refers to the perceived social pressure to perform or not to perform a behavior. The third one is the degree of perceived behavioral control, which refers to the perceived ease or difficulty of performing a behavior and it is assumed to reflect past experience as well as anticipated impediments and obstacles. As a general rule, the more favorable the attitude and subjective norm with respect to a behavior, and the greater the perceived behavioral control, the stronger should be an individual's intention to perform the behavior. (Ajzen, 2010; Noar & Zimmerman, 2005)

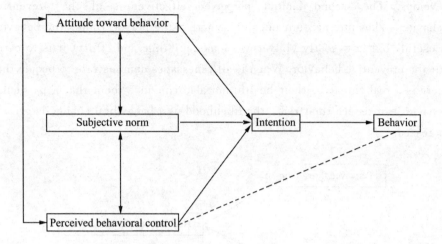

Figure 2-2   Theory of planned behavior

Many studies have found that TPB has improved the predictability of intention in various health-related fields such as leisure, exercise, diet, etc. (Ajzen, 1989; Ajzen & Driver, 1992; Albarracin et al., 2001; Conner, Kirk, Cade & Barrett, 2003; Nguyen, Potyin & Otis, 1997; Sheeran & Taylor, 2010) However, limitations are still claimed, TPB ignores individual needs and emotions, which can affect one's behavior, beliefs and other constructs of the model. (Sniehotta, 2010)

2.1.2.3   Health Belief Model

As one of the first theories of health behavior, Health Belief Model is a guideline to explain and describe the health-related behavior (Glanz & Bishop, 2010) It was developed in the 1950s by social psychologists at the US Public Health Service to better understand the widespread failure of screening programs for tuberculosis. (Carpenter, 2010; Glanz, Lewis & Rimer, 1997; Janz & Becker, 1984; Rosenstock, 1974)

As Figure 2-3 shows, HBM proposes that whether a person performs a particular health behavior is influenced by two major factors: the degree to which the disease (negative outcome) is perceived by the person as threatening, and the degree to which the health behavior is believed to be effective in reducing the risk of a negative health outcome. The first factor, perceived threat, is determined by whether someone believes he or she is susceptible to the disease, and how severe that person believes it would be if it develops. The second factor, perceived effectiveness of the preventive behavior, takes into account not only whether the person thinks the behavior is useful, but how costly (in terms of money, time and effort) it is to carry out the preventive behavior. When health messages demonstrate to people that there is a real threat to their health and also convince them that a particular behavior can reduce their risk, the likelihood of a behavioral change is greatly increased.

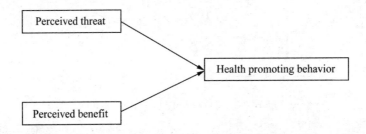

Figure 2-3　Health belief model

The HBM has been applied to predict a wide variety of health-related behaviors such as being screened for the early detection of asymptomatic diseases and receiving symptoms of diseases. More recently, the model has been applied to understand patient responses to symptoms of disease, compliance with medical regimens, and behaviors related to chronic illnesses. (Glanz et al., 1997, Rosenstock, Strecher & Becker, 1988; Strecher & Rosenstock, 1997)

However, the HBM has some limitations since it only accounts for individual differences in beliefs and attitudes, but not other factors that influence health behaviors, for instance, personal living habits. (smoking, drinking), environmental factors, economic factors, and emotional factors, etc. (Glanz et al., 1997; Janz & Becker, 1984)

2.1.2.4　Andersen Behavioral Model

Andersen Behavioral Model, which was developed by Ronald M. Andersen in 1968, is one of the most frequently used frameworks for the analysis of health care utilization. (Brown, Barner, Bohman & Richards, 2009; Eiman, Vilma & Adolfo, 2012; Glei, Goldman & Rodriguez, 2003; Kamgnia, 2006; Lopezcevallos & Chi, 2010; Najnin, Bennett & Luby, 2011;

Young et al., 2006)

　　As Figure 2-4 shows, this model assumes that the utilization of health care is influenced by the pre-disposition, the ability and the need to use health care services. (Andersen, 1995; Andersen & Newman, 2010)

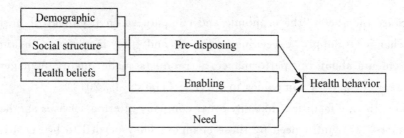

Figure 2-4　Andersen behavioral model

　　Pre-disposing factors related to the propensity to utilize health care services include individual characteristics that are not directly related to health care utilization but rather influence the likelihood of utilization. These characteristics can be categorized as demographic, social structure and health beliefs. Demographic characteristics include individual age and gender, which represent biological factors that affect the likelihood that an individual will need health care services. The social structure represents the factors that determine the status of an individual in the society as well as the physical, and social environment. The most common measures of social structure are education level, occupation and ethnicity. (Andersen, 1968) Health beliefs are the attitudes, values, and knowledge that an individual may have about health and health services that may influence utilization of health care services. (Andersen, 1995)

　　Enabling characteristics describe the means that individuals have at their disposal with which to utilize healthcare services. This is based on the argument that even though an individual may be pre-disposed to utilize health care services, certain factors must be in place to enable the actual use. These include income, health insurance status and availability of health care services. Usually residence (urban/rural) and distance are used as proxy measures for the availability of health services. (Andersen & Newman, 2010)

　　Need characteristics are the direct determinants of health care utilization, which include self-reported and evaluated morbidity. (Andersen & Newman, 2010)

2.2 Patient satisfaction

Since the 1980s, the economic and competitive environment of business has changed. Supply exceeding demand and the increasing customer's requirements about the performance of products made quality management become necessary for companies to survive. (Haj et al., 2013)

Health care facilities, like any other company offering services and having customers, were influenced by these changes. They needed to be sensitive to the needs and demands of patients. (Haj el al., 2013) Therefore, patient satisfaction has become an important indicator to evaluate the quality of care services provided by HCFs.

2.2.1 Definition of patient satisfaction

Although researches on patient satisfaction have been performed for several decades, the definition of patient satisfaction is quite difficult to be unified. (Carrhill, 2002) Previous studies have provided different definitions for patient satisfaction as follows:

Donabedian (1966) proposed that satisfaction was an outcome indicator according to the Donnebedian Model for evaluating the quality of care.

Pascoe (1983) deemed that satisfaction was an evaluation of the service directly received by the patient. It was the reaction of the health care recipient to the context, process, and result of the health care services.

Hall and Dornan (1988) stated that satisfaction was a multidimensional term that addressed, in addition to the care itself, other aspects such as access, quality, or cost.

Sitzia and Wood (1997) considered that patient satisfaction could be composed of determinants (i.e., patient characteristics and expectations) and components of satisfaction (i.e., interpersonal manner, outcomes of care, physical environment).

The American Nurse Association defined the patient satisfaction as measuring patient/family opinion regarding health care received from the nursing staff. This definition took into consideration the importance of the family feedback of patients about the delivered care. (Haj et al., 2013)

Speight (2005) regarded that patient satisfaction could be described as the extent of an individual experience compared with his or her expectations and the patient evaluation of the process of taking the medication and the outcomes associated with the medication. The patient attached values to specific attributes of the treatment or care service, and these were unique to each individual experience.

Brunero, Lamont and Fairbrother (2010) defined patient satisfaction as the extent to which treatment gratified the wants, wishes, and desires of the client for services.

Custer (2012) held that satisfaction referred generally to the match between expectations and real circumstances of the treatment. If expectations and service circumstances were equal, the client was generally satisfied; or conversely if the service circumstances fell below expectations, the client was dissatisfied. And the patient satisfaction was mostly linked to the interaction between physicians and patients, and then it exceeded that area to other domains of satisfaction.

From above we can see that patient satisfaction has been widely defined both as a process measure influencing other outcomes and an outcome measure after health care services.

As a process measure, studies have shown that patient satisfaction level can affect outcomes, such as their patterns of service utilization and treatment adherence over the course of their illness. Evidence suggested that satisfied patients were more likely to engage with health care services, adhere to therapy and get better results, while dissatisfied patients were at high risk of giving up treatments and facing adverse trajectories of health care. (Attkisson & Zwick, 1982; Lebow, 1983; Spensley, Edwards & White, 2010; Woodward, Berry & Bucci, 2017)

As an outcome measure, satisfaction has been described as the results of different factors, both at the patient and service level, such as the patient expectations of services, perceptions of the need for psychiatric care, and the patient-clinician relationship, as well as reflecting patient experience with health care services. (Henderson et al., 2010; Ruggeri et al., 2003, 2006;

Woodward et al., 2017)

Therefore, satisfaction is considered as an important source of quality of care received, and high satisfaction rating is increasingly pursued by health care professionals and service managers as an indicator of good service organization and delivery. (Cleary & McNeil, 1988; Edlund, Young, Kung, Sherbourne & Wells, 2010; Shipley et al., 2000)

2.2.2　Theories and models to evaluate patient satisfaction

Since researches on patient satisfaction have been performed for several decades, a plethora of theories and instruments measuring satisfaction have been developed. Introductions about these theories and instruments are as follows.

2.2.2.1　Discrepancy Theory of Satisfaction

The Discrepancy Theory of Satisfaction defines satisfaction as the difference between what is desired or needed and what is perceived to occur. It has been widely adopted to investigate the association between patient desires and satisfaction. For example, Like and Zyzanski (1987) found that the fulfillment of patient desires by physicians was strongly correlated with the visit satisfaction.

However, the Discrepancy Theory could not explain the variation in satisfaction very well. It assumes that any deviation from what is expected will create dissatisfaction, no matter the outcome is more negative or more positive than expected. Williams found that the variation explained by discrepancies between expectations and satisfaction, controlling for socio-demographic differences, remained at under 20%. (Williams, 1994)

2.2.2.2　Fulfillment Theory of Satisfaction

Fulfillment Theory focuses on outcome measures of health care. It is assumed that there is a direct relationship between fulfillment factors (outcome) and satisfaction, which means that if the fulfillment is related to satisfaction, one would expect a direct relationship between satisfaction and the outcomes of care, such as improved physical, mental, or social functioning. (Worthington, 2005)

With the theory, Covinskey et al. (2010) found that there was no association between health status change and satisfaction, once the baseline health status was controlled for; those with higher functioning or better outcomes would be more satisfied, no matter there was an improvement during the period of care or not.

However, the Fulfillment Theory is regarded logically inadequate, because the objective outcomes alone can determine satisfaction. (Worthington, 2005)

2.2.2.3 Consumer Models of Satisfaction

In 1983, Pascoe suggested that the consumer models of satisfaction might be incorporated into patient satisfaction modeling. (Pascoe, 1983) Below is the introduction of several commonly used consumer models.

The Contrast Theory suggests that when consumers perceive a difference between expectations and outcomes, they will magnify the difference. The Assimilation Theory suggests that when consumers perceive an inconsistency between expectations and outcomes, they will decrease or assimilate the inconsistency in order to adjust perceptions of outcomes to be consistent with expectations. (Pascoe, 1983; Festinger, 1957)

The combination of the two theories, the Assimilation-Contrast Theory, suggests that a consumer satisfaction response will be nonlinear, which means that assimilation will occur within a certain range of discrepancy between expectations and outcome (the zone of tolerance), while outside the range, the contrast effect will occur and inconsistencies will be magnified, leading to either dissatisfaction or higher satisfaction than within the assimilation range. (Pascoe, 1983)

Furthermore, Oliver (1993, 1997) incorporated the Fulfillment Theory, Discrepancy Theory, and Assimilation-Contrast theory in a model of consumer satisfaction, with an addition of the affect as an explicit component of this model. He suggested that satisfaction was partly a cognitive reaction and partly an affective reaction; and according to previous research results, affect was composed of both positive and negative dimensions, which operated simultaneously.

Consumer models of satisfaction, compared with previous models, acknowledge the complexity of the factors related to satisfaction. However, attempts to apply consumer models of satisfaction into the health care field have been only partially successful due to the multiple dimensions of health care services and cultural contexts. (Alden, Do & Bhawuk, 2004; Bowers, Swan & Koehler, 1994; Carman, 1990; Parasuraman, Zeithaml & Berry, 1988) Moreover, although consumer models address the emotional aspects of service reactions, they neglect the important relationship between health care professionals and patients, and other social contexts of health care. (Williams, 1994)

The notion of health care recipients as consumers in these models has also been challenged, which assumes that patients have bargaining power, freedom of choice, the knowledge and the motivation to choose a particular option from available services, and the power to challenge medical authority. However, studies found that these assumptions did not necessarily hold at the individual level. (Avis, Bond & Arthur, 1997; Dawson et al., 2002; Edwards Staniszewska & Crichton, 2010; Lupton, Donaldson & Lloyd, 1991; Lupton, 1997; Sinding, 2003; Williams, Coyle & Healy, 1998)

2.2.2.4 Sociological Perspective Theories of Satisfaction

As previous theories do not recognize the social contexts of health care or the social influences on health care recipients. Sociological Perspective Theories of Satisfaction were proposed to examine the interactional and social aspects of determinants of satisfaction. These theories assume that individual social contexts and the interpersonal and power relationships between health care professionals and patients must be incorporated into modeling, and the broader determinants of satisfaction (other than individual perceptions and attitudes) should be considered. (Annandale, 2014)

Compared with previous theories and models, the sociological perspective theories are more comprehensively and widely used methods for evaluating patient satisfaction.

2.2.3 Scales for measuring patient satisfaction

Derived from many theories and models of satisfaction, numerous measurement scales for patient satisfaction have been developed. These scales focus on various aspects of health care services, such as communication with health care providers, access to HCFs, the quality of basic amenities, waiting time to make an appointment and to receive health care services. (Bleich et al., 2009; Aletras et al., 2009) However, most of these instruments are specific to a country's health care system or type of HCFs, which make comparisons among countries and over time rather difficult. (Miglietta, Belessiotisrichards, Ruggeri & Priebe, 2018).

2.2.3.1   Client Satisfaction Questionnaire

The most commonly used measurement of patient satisfaction in studies was the Client Satisfaction Questionnaire (CSQ). (Larsen, Attkisson, Hargreaves & Nguyen, 1979) It was developed with a goal of building a standardized measure having strong psychometric properties that could be used to assess satisfaction with service across various types of health and human services.

The scales are now used worldwide in more than thirty languages. Different versions of CSQ vary in the number of questions included. For example, the eight-item version of this questionnaire measures general satisfaction, with items such as "Did you get the kind of service you wanted?" and "To what extent has our program met your needs?" Though the authors do not define their concepts of satisfaction, the items included in the final measure suggest satisfaction is the extent to which a service user considers their needs and wishes to have been met. (Woodward, Berry, & Bucci, 2017)

The CSQ has been adopted in quality assurance, evaluation research, and services research studies across a wide range of health care services, including outpatient and inpatient mental HCFs, public health center clinics, primary care health clinics, health maintenance organizations, patients with anorexia and bulimia, and so on.

2.2.3.2   Verona Service Satisfaction Scale

The Verona Service Satisfaction Scale (VSSS) was developed as a validated, multi-dimensional scale for measuring the satisfaction of patients with mental health services. (Knudsen et al., 2000)

The first 82-item version consisted of a set of 37 items cross-setting for health services and a set of 45 items specific for mental health services. The former group of items involves aspects meaning priorities across a broad array of health care setting, including overall satisfaction, professional skills and behavior and efficacy. The latter group of items involves aspects which are specifically relevant in mental health settings, particularly in community-based services, such as social skills and types of intervention. (Attkinson &

Greenfield, 1999; Greenfield & Attkinson, 1989; Ruggeri & Greenfield, 1995)

After confirming the acceptability, content validity, sensitivity, and reliability of the VSSS-82 (Ruggeri, 1994; Ruggeri & Dall'Agnola, 1993; Ruggeri, Dall'Agnola, Bisoffi & Greenfield, 1996), the intermediate (VSSS-54) and the short (VSSS-32) versions of VSSS were developed based on the VSSS-82, which could be used in the everyday clinical setting. So far, different versions of VSSS have been translated into various languages and applied in studies in many places all over the world. (Clarkson et al., 2010; Haycox, et al., 1999; Henderson et al., 1999; Leese et al., 1998; Merinder et al., 1999; Parkman et al., 1997)

2.2.3.3　Hospital Consumer Assessment of Health Care Providers and Systems

The Hospital Consumer Assessment of Health Care Providers and Systems (HCAHPS) survey was developed by the Centers for Medicare and Medicaid Services with the collaboration of the Agency for Health Quality Research in 2002. (Elliott et al., 2010; Elliott, Kanouse, Edwards & Hilborne, 2009; Giordano et al., 2010) So far, it has been the most known standardized and unbiased set of measures of patient experience in the USA. (Vogus & McClelland, 2016)

The HCAHPS survey measures the discharged inpatient experiences of the hospital care, employing 25 patient rating items with respect to the communication with nurses and doctors, the responsiveness of hospital staff, the cleanliness and quietness of hospital environment, pain management, communication about medicines, discharge information, overall rating of hospital, and willingness to recommend the hospital, as well as questions regarding patient demographics. (CMS, 2014)

The HCAHPS survey had been endorsed by the National Quality Forum in the USA, and it was also selected for the purposes of the European Commission RN4CAST project, which involved 12 countries (Belgium, England, Finland, Germany, Greece, Ireland, The Netherlands, Norway, Poland, Spain, Sweden and Switzerland) because of its potentiality to yield comparable results that would allow to obtain objective and meaningful comparisons across health systems on domains that are important to consumers among the participating European countries and the USA. (Squires et al., 2012)

2.2.3.4　Patient Judgment of Hospital Quality

The Patient Judgment of Hospital Quality (PJHQ) questionnaire was developed by Rubin, Meterko, Nelson,and Meterkoin in 1990.

The tool inquiries inpatient experience covering the overall satisfaction with received health care services, and five specific hospital practices, including admissions, nursing, and daily care, medical care, information, and hospital environment and ancillary staff. Also, questions concerning the prior and recent hospitalizations (number of prior hospitalizations, prior consultations, choice of hospital, self-reported condition at admission, need for assistance, etc.), recommendation of hospital to others, and intention to return to the same hospital are included.

2.2.4　Scale for measuring patient satisfaction in China

It can be seen from the above that most of the scales evaluating patient satisfaction are developed in English. Translating questionnaires may be inappropriate because satisfaction is closely dependent on the cultural background and health care systems. Before using a translated foreign questionnaire, it is necessary to perform a transcultural validation according to specific rules and methods. (Baider, Everhadani & Denour, 1995; Charles et al., 1994) As a result, it is preferable to use questionnaires devised in the country of origin. (Boyera, 2009)

In addition, most of these scales are originated in well-developed countries, and are specific to the health care system in a specific country. Unlike most of the developed countries, China has a special health care environment (scarce and unbalanced health care resources) and a large population. Therefore, directly applying these scales into studies carried out in our country may be not suitable.

So far, the only one large sample research regarding patient satisfaction in China is the National Health Services Survey (NHSS). Starting from 2003, the 3rd NHSS has begun the evaluations on patient satisfaction with only a few 3-point likert items, which could not fulfill a comprehensive measurement for patient satisfaction, and thus health care quality.

2.3　Knowledge gaps

A number of studies on patient HCSB and satisfaction have been carried out in China, which provided helpful evidences for policy design and improvement. However, there are still a number of knowledge gaps about inpatient HCSB and satisfaction, as well as relevant influential factors in rural backward areas, which must be distinguished from those in developed areas and urban areas, because the socio-economic development and local regulation and policy details vary greatly across the regions. Therefore, this study tries to fill the knowledge gaps in the following respects:

（1）Questionnaire design. On the basis of the NHSS, a more comprehensive questionnaire specialized in the evaluation on inpatient health care service is developed. Besides, a series of 5-point likert items measuring different aspects of patient satisfaction, questions regarding participant socio-demographic characteristics and reasons for their dissatisfaction are also inquired to investigate the influential factors for the inpatient satisfaction.

（2）Inpatient HCSB in rural western China. Besides the inpatient HCSB and the relevant factors in rural western China, the reasons for the inpatients choosing the corresponding HCFs are also explored in this study, which provides more intuitive information for the investigation of inpatient health care demands and the evaluation of the local health care quality. Moreover, combined with the analysis of the inpatient satisfaction and dissatisfaction, this study identifies the importance of a number of attributes associated with the inpatient HCSB and satisfaction, provides a more comprehensive and persuasive results of the inpatient preferences, needs and demands, as well as the inpatient health care quality in rural western China.

（3）Overall inpatient satisfaction evaluation. Besides the evaluation on satisfaction with each single aspect of the inpatient health care service, the overall inpatient satisfaction is measured with a model constructed by the exploratory factor analysis. With the model, the results of this study could be used as a baseline among areas and over time.

Chapter 3   Objective and methodology

Study objectives and research strategies are described in this chapter. Also, the detailed methods are provided for the specific objectives.

3.1   Research objectives

The general objective of this study is to investigate inpatient health care seeking behavior and satisfaction with inpatient health care services in rural western China, and to explore the relative internal and external influential factors. This study also attempts to provide some policy recommendations and suggestive strategies based on the results.

The specific objectives include:

(1) To investigate the inpatient choice of HCFs;

(2) To assess the reasons that patients adopted the corresponding HCFs;

(3) To identify factors that affected patient utilization of HCFs;

(4) To explore the inpatient satisfaction with each single aspect the inpatient care service that they received;

(5) To identify aspects that the inpatients were dissatisfied with about the health care services;

(6) To set a comprehensive model for evaluating the overall inpatient satisfaction;

(7) To determine factors associated with the inpatient satisfaction with the inpatient services that they received.

3.2　Research design

For the general objectives, a cross-sectional study involving multiple sites was employed in rural western China. And for each specific objective, the research design is as following:

For Objectives 1 and 2, descriptive analyses were applied to describe distribution, central tendency and dispersion. As there were many differences among different types of HCFs and in inpatient socio-economic status, Chi-square test was used to calculate differences between proportions, and t-test and one-way ANOVA was used to compare differences between means.

For Objective 3, by using the raw data and the results of the Objectives 1 and 2, a multinomial logistic regression was performed to explore the factors affecting inpatient HCSB, using main effects model and odds ration to indicate the association between these factors and patient choice. Before the multinomial logistic regression, a univariate analysis was applied, in which variables showed that statistical significance would be included in the multinomial logistic regression as independent variables.

For Objectives 4, 5 and 6, descriptive analyses were applied to describe distribution, and Chi-square test was used to compare differences in the inpatient satisfaction among different types of HCFs. To evaluate the overall inpatient satisfaction, an EFA was applied for multiple rank variables made study complicated. The EFA is a simple, well-developed and commonly used statistical method applied to examine the covariance relationship amongst a large number of observed items and to derive latent factors to account for these relationships.

For Objective 7, by using the raw data and the results of the Objectives 4, 5 and 6, a multiple linear regression was employed to identify the factors that had significant impacts on the inpatient satisfaction. In the multiple linear regression analysis, the overall inpatient satisfaction score was used as the dependent variable, and the proposed independent variables were the demographic characteristics of the inpatients (gender, age, education, career, income, health insurance, etc.) and characteristics of the specific HCFs (type and location).

To predict the acceptability and feasibility of the questionnaire, and to improve the design quality and efficiency, the pilot study was conducted with a small-size population.

Local reimbursement percentage, medical price, residents' income, education level and clinical opinions were further considered, and corresponding justifications were made after the pilot study.

3.3 Data source

Data was collected by undertaking several field surveys by our project team as well as some partnership organizations.

3.3.1 Field survey

Field surveys were carried out in rural western China to collect the empirical data related to the inpatient HCSB and satisfaction.

In 2014, except for Chongqing, eleven administrative areas in western China were recruited as study regions to carry out the field studies, including Ningxia Hui Autonomous Region, Guangxi Zhuang Autonomous Region, Xinjiang Weiwuer Autonomous Region, Gansu Province, Shaanxi Province, Sichuan Province, Guizhou Province, Yunnan Province, Qinghai Province, Inner Mongolia and Tibet Autonomous Region.

The planned criteria for selecting the sites of HCFs in each administrative area was to select three counties based on the discrepancy of economic development (GDP per capita): good, moderate and low, then to select three towns in each county with systematic sampling by ranking the towns with their population. Commonly, there was only one grassroot health institution for the inpatient health care services in each town, so the township hospital (TH) in each town was certainly selected. To ensure the sample size of the county-level HCFs in the research, in each county three county-level HCFs, including the county-level general hospital (CGH), the county-level traditional Chinese medicine hospital (CTCMH), and the county-level maternal and childcare hospital (CMCCH) were recruited in the study.

3.3.2 Literature and document review

Official documents from international health organizations, such as World

Health Organization (WHO), national documents and statistical yearbooks from National Health Commission of the People's Republic of China (NHC), and provincial documents from local health authorities were reviewed to fully understand the policy context and to obtain supporting data. Domestic and international peer-reviewed journals and research programs related to the research topic were also referenced.

3.4   Sampling and data collection

Considering that the average number of patients in county-level HCFs is higher than that in THs, 50 inpatients from each county-level HCFs and 30 ones from each TH were interviewed through a questionnaire. The total number of patients interviewed was 5,138, while the total number of the valid questionnaires was 4,050, and the effective rate was 78.9%. As shown in Table 3-1, among the valid respondents, 1,198 (29.6%) were from the CGHs, 785 (19.4%) were from the CTCMHs, 629 (15.5%) were from the CMCCHs, and the rest 1,438 (35.5%) were from the THs. The number of valid respondents varied in different autonomous areas, with the most in Sichuan, which was 710 (17.5%), and the least in Tibet, which was 107 (2.6%).

Table 3-1   **Number and distribution of valid participants**

	No. of participants				
	CGH	CTCMH	CMCCH	TH	Total
Yunnan	103	31	32	94	260
Inner Mongolia	176	83	27	0	286
Sichuan	145	160	136	269	710
Guangxi	104	98	132	162	496
Xinjiang	120	46	109	181	456
Gansu	124	86	43	258	511
Tibet	107	0	0	0	107
Guizhou	108	90	0	150	348
Shaanxi	110	74	38	47	269

Continued

	No. of participants				
	CGH	CTCMH	CMCCH	TH	Total
Qinghai	0	41	72	171	284
Ningxia	101	76	40	106	323
Total	1,198	785	629	1,438	4,050

3.5 Questionnaire design

The questionnaire (see Appendix I) consisted of two parts: the first part included questions regarding individual characteristics of the participants (e.g. age, gender, education level, career, insurance, income, whether having chronic diseases); the second part included 2 multiple-choice questions that account for choosing the HCF and for the dissatisfaction, and a series of 9 questions about satisfaction with every single aspect of the received inpatient health care services, including whether medical staffs clearly explaining disease conditions, whether being asked for the opinion on medical regimens, attitude of medical staffs, status of medical equipment, HCF environment, medical expenditures, level of technology, reliability of medical staffs, and the general satisfaction with the HCF. For each question, the degree of satisfaction was rated using a 5-point Likert item from 1 (very dissatisfied) to 5 (very satisfied).

With informed and written consent, all the participating patients filled the questionnaire independently. The questionnaire background and all questions were explained by trained investigators. The questionnaires for interviewees under 14 were answered by their adult guardians. And all the data were kept confidential just for this study and were not revealed or discussed with other people.

3.6 Data processing and analysis

By using Microsoft Office Excel 2013, quantitative and qualitative data were typed in and double checked by two individual members of our team, and then coded and organized for cleaning to ensure there were no errors and omissions. IBM SPSS version 21.0 was applied for the statistical interpretation and statistical inference.

Descriptive statistics for distribution, central tendency and dispersion were calculated. Chi-square test was used to calculate differences between proportions, and t-test and one-way ANOVA were used to compare differences between means. Univariate analysis and multivariate regressions were used to investigate the influential factors of patient HCSB and satisfaction. Results with a 2-sided p value <0.05 were considered statistically significant.

3.6.1 Methods for determining the influential factors of inpatient HCSB

A multinomial logistic regression was performed to explore the factors affecting the inpatient HCSB, using main effects model and odds ration to indicate the association between these factors and patient choices.

Before the multinomial analysis, a univariate analysis was performed. Since this was an exploratory study, variables with a p value no more than 0.3 in the univariate analysis would be included in the multinomial logistic regression as the independent variables, and the inpatient choice of HCFs was included as the dependent variable.

Drawing from the Andersen Health Model, independent variables applied in this study included predisposing, enabling and need characteristics of individuals. Predisposing characteristics included age, gender, education level, and career. Enabling characteristics included income, health insurance. For the need characteristics, self-reported chronic illness was recruited. Moreover, reasons for the inpatients choosing the specific HCF were also included in the analysis.

3.6.2 Methods used to evaluate the overall inpatient satisfaction

The EFA was applied to measure the overall satisfaction of the inpatients with the health care services that they received.

The EFA is a statistical method used to examine the covariance relationship among a large number of observed items and to derive latent factors to account for these relationships. (Mulaik, 2009; Field, 2009). The goal of EFA is to reduce the dimensionality of the original space and to give an interpretation to the new space, sanned by a reduced number of new dimensions which are supposed to underlie the old ones (Rietveld & van Hout 1993), or to explain the variance in the observed variables in terms of underlying latent factors (Habing, 2003). Thus, EFA offers not only the possibility of gaining a clear view of the data, but also the possibility of using the output in subsequent analyses. (Field 2000; Rietveld & van Hout 1993)

The appropriateness of the factor model was examined prior to using the EFA by the Barlett's test and the Kaiser-Meyer-Olkin (KMO) test. The Barlett's test is based on the null hypothesis of no correlation between items, and a significant test result implies that sufficient correlation exists among the items. (Bartlett, 1954) The KMO measures sampling adequacy for the execution of the EFA. Its value ranges from 0 to 1; the higher the value, the stronger the correlation between items. (Kaiser, 1974; Norusis, 1993) The KMO value should be 0.6 or higher for a satisfactory EFA to proceed. (Tabachnick & Fidell, 2007; Kaiser, 1974)

Moreover, the internal consistency of a group of items was assessed by the Cronbach's alpha test. (Cronbach, 1951) It was suggested that a Cronbach's alpha value of 0.7 or higher could be considered to have a high consistency, the value between 0.35 and 0.7 is moderately reliable, and the value less than 0.35 is not acceptable. (Guilford, 1965) Bradley (1994) deemed that the lowest Cronbach's alpha value indicating adequate consistency increases with the number of items. For instance, for a three-item scale, a value of 0.5 was adequate, while for a ten-item scale, the value should be greater than 0.7.

Principal component factor extraction with a Varimax (orthogonal) rotation was used to identify meaningful components. The number of latent factors to be retained could be determined by using the Kaiser rule (Kaiser, 1960) and scree cut-off points (Cattell, 1966). The extraction communality of an item estimated the proportion of the variance in each variable accounted for by the factor solutions. (Rietveld & van Hout, 1993) Large extraction communality values indicated that the items within each domain had a very high association among them. All extraction communalities were restricted to be higher than 0.5. (Field, 2009; Stevens, 1992)

In this study, a Cronbach's alpha test was run firstly to measure the internal consistency of the 9 single aspects to see whether they all reliably assessed the inpatient satisfaction. Then an EFA was conducted to extract the appropriate number of factors (representing different sub-domains of the inpatient satisfaction), obtain all item loadings on each factor, and extract factor score coefficients of all items. The score of each factor was a summation of the factor score coefficient of each item multiplied to their corresponding scores. The weight of each factor was equal to the percentage of the variance that it explained. And the score for the overall inpatient satisfaction was a linear aggregation of the weighted sums of all factor scores.

For each satisfaction factor, the value was computed using：

$$OSI_{ij} = \sum_{k=1}^{n} w_{kj} I_k$$

Where OS was an index for the satisfaction factor j, and w_{kj} denoted the weight of satisfaction indicator k in the satisfaction factor j and I_k represented the value of the satisfaction indicator k. The weights w_{kj} were computed from the varimax rotation as follows：

$$W_{kj} = \frac{(factorloading)^2}{eigenvalue_j}$$

3.6.3 Methods for exploring the influential factors of the inpatient satisfaction

After the overall satisfaction was determined, a multiple linear regression was employed to identify the factors that had significant impacts on the inpatient satisfaction. In the multiple linear regression, the overall inpatient satisfaction score was used as the dependent variable, and the proposed independent variables were the demographic characteristics of the inpatients (gender, age, education, career, income, health insurance, etc.) and characteristics of the corresponding HCFs (type and location).

3.7 Data quality assurance

The completeness, consistency and clarity of data were assured by quality control mechanisms throughout all phases of data collection, entry, and analysis.

Prior to data collection, all data collectors were well trained in data collection skills and ethical approach, including confidentiality.

During field survey, data collectors clearly explained the purpose of investigations. Completed questionnaires were checked on the spot, and any missing questions or errors were corrected by returning to the respondents when possible.

During the data entry, all the data was double checked by two individuals of the research team. The questionnaires including discrepancies or errors that could not be corrected were excluded.

Chapter 4　Result I: Inpatient health care seeking behavior

This chapter presents the results of inpatient health care seeking behaviors in rural western China, factors influencing the behaviors, and how the behaviors were influenced.

4.1　Demographic characteristics of the inpatients

As is shown in Table 4-1, for the participating inpatients in different types of HCFs, the compositions including gender, age, education level, occupation, monthly income, health insurance, and chronic disease were significant different.

Among all the participants, 42.9% were male and 57.1% were female. However, in the CMCCHs, the percentage of female inpatients was much higher than those in the other types of HCFs, which was 79.7%.

As for age, the inpatients between 25 and 34 years old accounted for the biggest proportion at 21.4%; and those less than 14 years old accounted for the smallest proportion at 3.1%. And in the CMCCH, the participants between 25 and 34 years old took up a much higher proportion at 44.5%, and the proportion of the participants above 45 years old were much lower than those in the other types of HCFs.

In terms of the education level, the participants with an elementary school degree or a middle school degree made up the highest proportions, which corresponded to 28.2% and 28.6%, respectively; the participants with a degree of college and above made up the lowest proportion, which corresponded to 12. 2%. However, in the CMCCHs, compared with the other three types of HCFs, the proportions of the illiterate inpatients and inpatients with an elementary school degree were relatively lower, which were 6. 7% and 14. 8%, respectively; and the proportion of the inpatients with a middle school or a high school degree were relatively higher, which were 36. 1% and 24. 6%, respectively. And in the THs, the proportions of the illiterate inpatients and inpatients with an elementary school degree were comparatively higher, which were 20. 4% and 35. 5%, respectively; and the proportion of the inpatients with a degree of high school or college and above were comparatively lower, which were 10. 7% and 6. 7%, respectively.

As regards the occupation, farmers accounted for the largest proportion, which was 49. 1%. But the proportion of farmers was comparatively lower in the CMCCHs (30. 2%), and comparatively higher in the THs (65. 0%).

And most participants had a monthly income of no more than 2,000 *yuan*; 31. 3% had no income and 43. 8% had a monthly income of 1-2,000 *yuan*. The proportions of the inpatients with a monthly income of more than 2,000 *yuan* were larger in the county-level HCF than in the THs.

Moreover, 70. 1% of the participating inpatients had enrolled in the NRCMS, which occupied the greatest proportion. However, in THs the proportion of the inpatients insured by the NRCMS was even higher at 84. 4%, and correspondingly the proportions of the inpatients insured by the UEBMI (Urban employee Basic Medical Insurance) and URBMI were lower than those in the county-level HCFs.

And 27. 8% of the interviewed inpatients suffered from chronic diseases, while the proportion in the CMCCHs was relatively lower at 12. 7%.

Table 4-1   **Demographic characteristics of the inpatients**

		CGH	CTCMH	CMCCH	TH	Total
Gender***	Male	48.1%	46.0%	20.3%	46.7%	42.9%
	Female	51.9%	54.0%	79.7%	53.3%	57.1%
Age***	≤14	2.3%	3.8%	4.3%	2.9%	3.1%
	15-24	11.8%	7.5%	20.3%	7.9%	10.9%
	25-34	21.2%	14.1%	44.5%	15.5%	21.4%
	35-44	18.3%	17.5%	16.5%	17.2%	17.5%

Continued

		CGH	CTCMH	CMCCH	TH	Total
Age***	45-54	17.9%	19.6%	8.6%	18.2%	16.9%
	55-64	13.6%	19.4%	3.8%	18.8%	15.1%
	≥65	14.9%	18.1%	1.9%	19.5%	15.1%
Education level***	Illiteracy	14.9%	12.9%	6.7%	20.4%	15.2%
	Elementary school	25.9%	29.0%	14.8%	35.5%	28.2%
	Middle school	26.9%	28.9%	36.1%	26.6%	28.6%
	High school	16.3%	17.2%	24.6%	10.7%	15.8%
	College and above	16.0%	12.0%	17.8%	6.7%	12.2%
Occupation***	Farmer	43.5%	43.8%	30.2%	65.0%	49.1%
	Worker	7.9%	8.9%	12.6%	9.6%	9.4%
	Business/Service	11.0%	10.7%	15.3%	7.0%	10.2%
	Teacher/Government staff	15.2%	14.4%	14.9%	5.1%	11.4%
	Student	5.5%	3.9%	5.9%	3.8%	4.7%
	Retired	4.1%	5.4%	0.6%	1.9%	3.0%
	Others	12.8%	12.9%	20.5%	7.6%	12.1%
Monthly income***	None	28.9%	31.3%	28.6%	34.6%	31.3%
	1-2,000	43.2%	41.5%	42.3%	46.2%	43.8%
	2,001-4,000	21.5%	23.1%	24.8%	15.8%	20.3%
	4,000 and above	6.5%	4.1%	4.3%	3.4%	4.6%
Health insurance***	National health insurance	3.8%	4.2%	1.6%	1.3%	2.6%
	UEBMI	16.3%	15.5%	14.9%	4.9%	11.9%
	URBMI	9.5%	9.8%	8.3%	4.7%	7.7%
	NRCMS	61.6%	61.8%	63.8%	84.4%	70.1%
	URRMI	3.4%	3.8%	3.7%	1.8%	3.0%
	Others	1.4%	1.0%	1.3%	0.9%	1.1%
	None	4.0%	3.8%	6.5%	1.9%	3.6%
Chronic disease***	Yes	28.4%	29.4%	12.7%	33.0%	27.8%
	No	71.6%	70.6%	87.3%	67.0%	72.2%

*** $p < 0.001$

4.2 Reasons for inpatients choosing HCFs

The multiple-choice question was applied to investigate reasons why the interviewed inpatients chose the corresponding HCFs. An average of 2.05 options was given by each patient.

The results exhibited in Table 4-2 and Figure 4-1 show that "convenient location" "reasonable charge" "good service attitude" and "professional quality" were the four reasons of most concerns. However, for interviewees from different types of HCFs, the focus points varied.

In the CGHs, the four reasons with the most concern were, in descending order, "convenient location" "good service attitude" "professional quality" and "reasonable charge". In the CTCMHs, the four reasons were "good service attitude" "reasonable charge" "convenient location" and "professional quality" in descending order. In the CMCCHs, the four reasons were "convenient location" "reasonable charge" "good service attitude" and "professional quality" in descending order. And in the THs, the four reasons were "convenient location" "reasonable charge" "good service attitude" and "professional quality" in descending order.

Table 4-2   Reasons for inpatients choosing HCFs

	GH	TCMH	MCCH	TH	Total
Convenient location	51.7%	39.1%	40.0%	63.7%	51.7%
Reasonable charge	31.8%	41.5%	35.3%	35.6%	35.6%
Professional quality	35.6%	34.3%	27.7%	19.6%	28.4%
Advanced equipment	22.7%	20.0%	16.1%	10.8%	16.9%
Sufficient drug supply	8.1%	9.0%	6.8%	6.1%	7.4%
Good service attitude	37.7%	41.9%	35.2%	26.3%	34.1%
Designated HCF	15.3%	13.5%	14.7%	15.0%	14.7%
Having trusted doctors	14.3%	16.9%	12.4%	12.7%	13.9%
Having acquaintance	6.3%	9.9%	6.0%	3.4%	5.9%

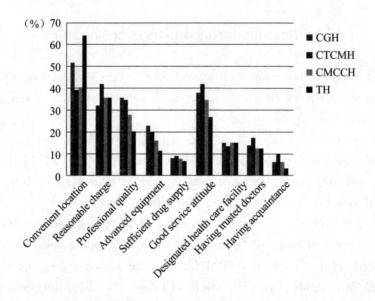

Figure 4-1   Reasons for inpatients choosing HCFs

4.3   Influential factors of the inpatient HCSB

The results of the univariate logistic regression are presented in Table 4-3. Except for "designed HCFs", all the other factors with a p value of no more than 0.3 were recruited into the following multinomial logistic regress analysis to explore the factors that influenced patient health care seeking behavior.

Table 4-3   **Results of the univariate logistic regression[a]**

Variables	-2 Log Likelyhood	DF	p
Province	157.410	30	0.000***
Gender	44.772	3	0.000***
Age	126.276	18	0.000***
Education level	97.482	12	0.000***
Occupation	123.037	18	0.000***
Monthly income	78.618	9	0.000***

Continued

Variables	-2LogLikelyhood	DF	p
Health insurance	112.518	18	0.000***
Chronic disease status	44.091	3	0.000***
Convenient location	45.024	3	0.000***
Reasonable charge	44.914	3	0.001**
Professional qualities	44.503	3	0.000***
Advanced equipment	43.370	3	0.000***
Sufficient drug supply	41.281	3	0.073+
Good service attitude	44.849	3	0.000***
Designated HCF	43.057	3	0.656
Trusted doctors	42.955	3	0.051+
Acquaintance	40.659	3	0.000***

** $p < 0.01$, *** $p < 0.001$, + $p < 0.3$.

a: The reference category is township hospitals.

The results of the multinomial logistic regression were shown in Table 4-4. The odds ratio (OR) and p value indicate that factors having effects on the inpatient HCSB included province, gender, age, occupation, monthly income, health insurance, chronic disease status, and whether the HCF had a great location, reasonable charge, professional quality, advanced equipment, sufficient drug supply, good service attitude, and acquaintances.

In Inner Mongolia and Shaanxi, the interviewed inpatients preferred the county-level HCFs rather than the THs. In Inner Mongolia, the inpatients chose to visit the CTCMHs first (OR $= 1.062 \times 10^9$, $p = 0.000$), then the CGHs (OR $= 8.756 \times 10^8$, $p = 0.000$). In Shaanxi, the inpatients chose to go to the CTCMHs first (OR $= 4.275$, $p = 0.000$), then the CMCCHs (OR $= 3.072$, $p = 0.000$), and finally the CGHs (OR $= 2.394$, $p = 0.000$). In Sichuan (OR $= 0.377$, $p = 0.000$), Guangxi (OR $= 0.511$, $p = 0.001$), Xinjiang (OR $= 0.515$, $p = 0.001$), Gansu (OR $= 0.382$, $p = 0.000$), Guizhou (OR $= 0.527$, $p = 0.002$), the interviewees preferred the THs rather than the CGHs. And in Ningxia, the interviewees would like to visit the CTCMHs rather than the THs (OR $= 2.315$, $p = 0.003$).

Compared to the females, the male inpatients would like to visit the THs rather than the CMCCHs (OR=0.371, p=0.000).

Compared with the interviewees who were more than 65 years old, the younger inpatients tended to choose the CMCCHs rather than the THs. And the tendency roughly decreased with the growth of the age (for the inpatients younger than 15 years old, OR=14.471, p=0.000; for the inpatient between 15 and 24 years old, OR=11.756, p=0.000; for the inpatients between 25 and 34 years old, OR=15.124, p=0.000; for the inpatients between 35 and 44 years old, OR=6.864, p=0.000; for the inpatients between 45 and 54 years old, OR=4.922, p=0.000; for the inpatients between 55 and 64 years old, OR=2.432, p=0.000).

The inpatients with different occupations also had different preferences for HCFs. The farmers (for CGHs, OR=0.467, p=0.000; for CTCMHs, OR=0.498, p=0.000; for CMCCHs, OR=0.324, p=0.000), and the workers (for CGHs, OR=0.606, p=0.000; for CMCCHs, OR=0.533, p=0.000) preferred the THs rather than the county-level HCFs. And the students also showed a preference for the THs, compared to the CMCCHs (OR=0.327, p=0.000).

Compared with the inpatients with a monthly income of more than 4,000 *yuan*, the inpatients with no regular monthly income preferred the CTCMHs (OR=2.497, p=0.002) and the CMCCHs (OR=1.908, p=0.048) rather than the THs; and the inpatients with a monthly income less than 2,000 *yuan* preferred the CTCMHs rather than the THs (OR=1.879, p=0.022).

And taking respondents with no health insurance as the reference, the inpatients enrolled in the NRCMS would like to visit the THs firstly, the CTCMs secondly (OR=0.511, p=0.021), the CGHs thirdly (OR=0.451, p=0.003), and finally the CMCCHs (OR=0.323, p=0.000). While the inpatients having free medical care (FMC) (OR=0.342, p=0.000) and other types of health care insurance (OR=0.278, p=0.000) would like to visit the THs rather than the CMCCHs.

Compared with the respondents without chronic diseases, the inpatients suffering from chronic diseases preferred to visit the THs rather than the CGHs (OR=0.810, p=0.048) and the CMCCHs (OR=0.461, p=0.000).

For the inpatients who concerned the convenient locations when choosing

HCF, the THs were their primary choice, then the CGHs (OR=0.675, p=0.000) and the CMCCHs (OR=0.441, p=0.000), and the CTCMHs (OR=0.412, p=0.000) were their last choice.

For the inpatients who concerned the professional quality of medical staffs and advanced equipment in HCF, they preferred the CGHs (OR=1.909, p=0.000) and the CTCMs (OR=1.304, p=0.000) rather than the THs.

For the inpatients who cared about the sufficient drug supply, they would like to visit the THs rather than the CGHs (OR=0.626, p=0.000).

For the inpatients who cared about the service attitude of medical staff, they preferred the county-level HCFs rather than the THs (for CGHs, OR=1.462, p=0.000; for CTCMHs, OR=1.662, p=0.000; for CMCCHs, OR=1.693, p=0.000).

However, for the inpatients having the acquaintance in HCFs, they would like to go to the CTCMs rather than the THs (OR=2.307, p=0.000).

Table 4-4　　　Results of the multinomial logistic regression

	CGH[a]			CTCMH[a]		
	OR	95% CI	p	OR	95% CI	p
Province (reference=Yunnan)						
Inner Mongolia	8.756×10^8	$4.707 \times 10^8 -$ 1.629×10^9	0.000***	1.062×10^9	$5.226 \times 10^8 -$ 2.157×10^9	0.000***
Sichuan	0.377	0.255-0.558	0.000***	1.059	0.648-1.729	0.820
Ningxia	0.937	0.600-1.462	0.773	2.315	1.332-4.025	0.003**
Guangxi	0.511	0.342-0.764	0.001**	1.375	0.831-2.277	0.215
Xinjiang	0.515	0.344-0.769	0.001**	0.555	0.320-0.965	0.037*
Gansu	0.382	0.258-0.564	0.000***	0.734	0.442-1.216	0.230
Tibet	6.644×10^9	$0.000 - ^b$	0.997	2.548	$0.000 - ^b$	1.000
Guizhou	0.527	0.349-0.795	0.002**	1.174	0.702-1.964	0.540
Shaanxi	2.394	1.494-3.838	0.000***	4.275	2.407-7.594	0.000***
Qinghai	5.497×10^{-10}	$0.000 - ^b$	0.994	0.608	0.345-1.073	0.086
Gender (reference=female)						
Male	1.085	0.899-1.309	0.395	0.894	0.732-1.091	0.270

Continued

	CGH[a]			CTCMH[a]		
	OR	95% CI	*p*	OR	95% CI	*p*
Age (reference≥65)						
≤14	0.816	0.432-1.542	0.531	1.440	0.762-2.725	0.262
15-24	1.430	0.934-2.189	0.100	0.819	0.511-1.311	0.405
25-34	1.230	0.862-1.754	0.254	0.743	0.505-1.091	0.129
35-44	1.265	0.896-1.786	0.182	0.977	0.678-1.407	0.899
45-54	1.416	1.018-1.969	0.039*	1.407	1.001-1.977	0.049*
55-64	1.092	0.790-1.508	0.595	1.348	0.975-1.863	0.071
Education level (reference=college and above)						
Illiterate	0.894	0.548-1.460	0.655	0.872	0.512-1.486	0.615
Elementary	0.857	0.552-1.332	0.494	0.974	0.603-1.575	0.916
Middle school	1.033	0.688-1.550	0.876	1.297	0.832-2.023	0.251
High school	1.134	0.760-1.692	0.539	1.344	0.868-2.082	0.185
Occupation (reference=others)						
Farmer	0.467	0.339-0.643	0.000***	0.498	0.353-0.702	0.000***
Worker	0.606	0.392-0.936	0.024*	0.742	0.468-1.175	0.203
Business/ Service	1.103	0.711-1.712	0.661	1.232	0.768-1.975	0.387
Teacher/ Government staff	1.127	0.682-1.864	0.641	1.346	0.786-2.307	0.279
Student	0.660	0.372-1.168	0.154	0.541	0.286-1.025	0.060
Retired	1.002	0.528-1.902	0.995	1.390	0.710-2.720	0.336
Monthly income (reference=4,000 and above)						
None	1.521	0.916-2.526	0.105	2.497	1.400-4.456	0.002**
1-2,000	1.308	0.819-2.090	0.261	1.879	1.093-3.230	0.022*
2,001-4,000	1.008	0.630-1.611	0.975	1.574	0.919-2.696	0.099

Continued

	CGH[a]			CTCMH[a]		
	OR	95% CI	*p*	OR	95% CI	*p*
Health insurance (reference＝No insurance)						
FMC	0.814	0.354-1.872	0.628	1.103	0.467-2.609	0.823
UEBMI	1.529	0.814-2.873	0.187	1.524	0.779-2.982	0.218
URBMI	1.126	0.605-2.095	0.707	1.138	0.589-2.201	0.700
NRCMS	0.451	0.264-0.770	0.003**	0.511	0.289-0.904	0.021*
URRMI	1.013	0.464-2.213	0.975	1.522	0.688-3.364	0.300
Others	0.983	0.373-2.588	0.972	0.862	0.291-2.554	0.789
Chronic illness (reference＝No)						
Yes	0.810	0.657-0.998	0.048*	0.821	0.660-1.022	0.077
Convenient location (reference＝No)						
Yes	0.675	0.560-0.813	0.000***	0.412	0.338-0.502	0.000***
Reasonable charge (reference＝No)						
Yes	0.652	0.527-0.806	0.000***	1.088	0.877-1.350	0.443
Professional qualities (reference＝No)						
Yes	1.909	1.529-2.382	0.000***	1.304	1.030-1.650	0.027*
Advanced equipment (reference＝No)						
Yes	2.169	1.657-2.839	0.000***	1.450	1.085-1.937	0.012*
Sufficient drug supply (reference＝No)						
Yes	0.626	0.429-0.913	0.015*	0.834	0.563-1.235	0.365
Good service attitude (reference＝No)						
Yes	1.462	1.181-1.809	0.000***	1.662	1.332-2.073	0.000***
Having trusted doctor (reference＝No)						
Yes	1.084	0.826-1.421	0.562	1.235	0.936-1.629	0.136

Continued

	CGH[a]			CTCMH[a]		
	OR	95% CI	p	OR	95% CI	p
Having acquaintance (reference=No)						
Yes	1.430	0.924-2.212	0.108	2.307	1.523-3.494	0.000***

$*p<0.05$, $**p<0.01$, $***p<0.001$.

a：The reference category is township hospitals. b：Floating point overflow occurred while computing this statistic. Its value is therefore set to system missing.

Table 4-4   Results of the multinomial logistic regression (continued)

	CMCCH[a]		
	OR	95% CI	p
Province (reference=Yunnan)			
Inner Mongolia	$4.801×10^8$	$4.801×10^8$	
Sichuan	1.337	0.792-2.256	0.276
Ningxia	1.461	0.783-2.728	0.233
Guangxi	1.823	1.090-3.049	0.022*
Xinjiang	1.681	0.991-2.853	0.054
Gansu	0.448	0.252-0.798	0.006**
Tibet	2.639	0.000—[b]	1.000
Guizhou	$1.903×10^{-9}$	0.000—[b]	0.994
Shaanxi	3.072	1.607-5.873	0.001**
Qinghai	1.556	0.891-2.716	0.120
Gender (reference=female)			
Male	0.371	0.288-0.479	0.000***
Age (reference≥65)			
≤14	17.471	7.249-42.111	0.000***
15-24	11.756	5.766-23.966	0.000***
25-34	15.124	7.738-29.561	0.000***
35-44	6.864	3.462-13.607	0.000***
45-54	4.922	2.459-9.852	0.000***

Continued

	OR	CMCCH[a] 95% CI	p
55-64	2.432	1.164-5.081	0.018*
Education level (reference=college and above)			
Illiterate	0.722	0.390-1.336	0.299
Elementary	0.697	0.416-1.168	0.171
Middle school	1.263	0.803-1.988	0.312
High school	1.326	0.855-2.055	0.207
Occupation (reference=others)			
Farmer	0.324	0.224-0.470	0.000***
Worker	0.533	0.331-0.857	0.009**
Business/Service	0.731	0.451-1.187	0.205
Teacher/Government staff	0.737	0.422-1.290	0.285
Student	0.327	0.175-0.610	0.000***
Retired	0.666	0.203-2.185	0.503
Monthly income (reference=4,000 and above)			
None	1.908	1.006-3.619	0.048*
1-2,000	1.629	0.904-2.934	0.104
2,001-4,000	1.333	0.741-2.397	0.337
Health insurance (reference=No insurance)			
National health insurance	0.342	0.123-0.947	0.039*
UEBMI	0.626	0.312-1.255	0.187
URBMI	0.554	0.275-1.113	0.097
NRCMS	0.323	0.180-0.577	0.000***
URRMI	0.654	0.279-1.534	0.329
Others	0.278	0.091-0.848	0.024*
Chronic illness (reference=No)			
Yes	0.461	0.342-0.622	0.000***

Continued

		CMCCH[a]	
	OR	95% CI	p
Convenient location (reference=No)			
Yes	0.441	0.351-0.554	0.000***
Reasonable charge (reference=No)			
Yes	1.080	0.844-1.383	0.541
Professional qualities (reference=No)			
Yes	1.285	0.976-1.692	0.074
Advanced equipment (reference=No)			
Yes	1.217	0.870-1.702	0.251
Sufficient drug supply (reference=No)			
Yes	0.820	0.518-1.299	0.397
Good service attitude (reference=No)			
Yes	1.693	1.314-2.182	0.000***
Having trusted doctor (reference=No)			
Yes	0.906	0.648-1.266	0.563
Having acquaintance (reference=No)			
Yes	1.193	0.717-1.985	0.496

$^*p<0.05$, $^{**}p<0.01$, $^{***}p<0.001$.

a: The reference category is township hospitals. b: Floating point overflow occurred while computing this statistic. Its value is therefore set to system missing.

4.4 Discussion

Patient HCSB is an important and commonly used indicator for health care providers and payers to evaluate patient health care demand and health care service quality. Research on patient HCSB and its determinants can provide a scientific basis for the allocation of health care resources. Although several empirical researches have been completed to analyze the patient health care utilization in China, no large-scale intensive study specialized in the inpatient HCSB was performed.

In the current study, the inpatient HCSB in 11 provinces of the rural western China was analyzed. A total of 5,138 participants completed the survey questionnaire, the number of the valid questionnaires is 4,050, and the effective rate was 78.9%. Among the valid respondents, 35.5% were from the THs, and the rest were from the county-level HCFs, including 29.6% from the CGHs, 19.4% from the CTCMHs, and 15.5% from the CMCCHs.

Among all the valid respondents, 42.9% were male and 57.1% were female. This was consistent with the result of the 2013 NHSS report that female had a higher admission rate than male, and in rural western China, the rates were 11.2% and 7.6%, respectively. This might be due to the different physiological conditions and health care needs of male and female. (Cronbach, 1951; Guilford & Fruchter, 1973; Pinkhasov et al., 2010) Previous studies in Canada and the United States also found that for female, the chances of inpatient care utilization was 1.78 and 2.86 times of those for male. (Blackwell et al., 2009) And in the CMCCHs, 79.7% of the respondents were female, while the rest 20.3% were male. This was because that one of the most important responsibilities of the CMCCHs was to provide health care for women.

Except in the CMCCHs, there were no apparent differences among the age compositions of the respondents in the other 3 types of HCFs. In the CMCCHs, the proportion of respondents between 15 and 24 years old was 20.3%, and the proportion between 25 and 34 years old accounted for 44.5%, which was higher than those in the other 3 types of HCFs. The possible reason was that in the rural areas, the CMCCHs were the primary institutions providing health care for women of child bearing age.

The respondents with a higher education or a higher income level accounted for larger proportions in the county-level HCFs than in the THs, indicating that the patients with a higher education or income level were more likely to select higher level HCFs, and suggesting that patients with higher socioeconomic status would have better disease recognition ability and greater health care demand. The similar trend was observed in previous studies in both urban and rural areas. (Jia, 2010; Li, Wang, Liu & Sun, 2016; Wang et al, 2014; Yu, Zhao & Peng, 2006) Furthermore, compared with the county-level HCFs, the THs had a higher reimbursement rate and a lower minimum deductible. So for, the patients with a lower socioeconomic status may give priority to the THs when they selected health care provider. (Bartlett, 1954)

Compared with the county-level HCFs, the proportion of farmers was higher in the THs. This disclosed that farmers would like to choose the lower-level health care providers, while non-farmers were more likely to visit the higher-level health care providers. To some extent, the results also reflected that patients with higher socioeconomic status would pay more attention to health care quality, while patients of lower socioeconomic status would attach greater importance to health care expense. And on the other hand, this may be because more farmers are living in the towns than in the county district. For them, going to the THs are much more convenient. This was in according with the top reason for the inpatients choosing the corresponding HCFs, which was"convenient location".

The proportions of the inpatients enrolled in the UEBMI were greater in the county-level HCFs. In contrast, the proportion of the inpatients insured by the NRCMS was larger in the THs. The results were consistent with previous studies and revealed that the type of health insurance would influence patient health care seeking behavior (Wang, Zhang & Hou, 2016; Zhang, 2013; Zhao, Lang & Chang, 2015). And it might be due to the fact that the inpatients preferred a convenient location when choosing HCFs, and in the county district there were more residents insured by the UEBMI, while in the town there were more residents insured by the NRCMS.

And in the CMCCHs, the proportion of the patients suffering from chronic diseases was lower than those in the other 3 types of HCFs. The smaller proportion was probably because the chief responsibility of the CMCCH was to provide prevention and treatment for women and children.

The multiple-choice question survey showed how patients chose HCFs. "Convenient location" was the reason with top concern, followed by "reasonable charge" "service attitude" and "professional quality". The results were basically consistent with the previous studies in both urban and rural areas. (Bao et al., 2010; Chen et al. 2012; Duan, Pan & Ren, 2016; Gu, Yin & Qian, 2017; Guo, 2014; Yan, 2016; Yu et al., 2006) However, "Whether there is sufficient drug supply" or "whether there is acquaintance" were the two reasons with the least concern. This result was also consistent with the previous study, which stated that due to the information asymmetry, rural patients might not care much about the drug supply by generally following doctor's instruction on medications. (Jia, 2010)

Furthermore, the multinomial logistic analysis indicated that compared with the patients in the THs, the patients in the county-level HCFs had fewer concerns about the HCF location, but more concerns about the service attitude of medical staffs. And also in comparison with the patients in the THs, the patients in the CGHs cared more about the professional quality of medical staffs and medical equipment, but cared less about health care expense and the drug supply; the patients in the CTCMHs paid more attention to the professional quality of medical staffs, medical equipment and whether having an acquaintance. The results were in accordance with the former study. (Shan, 2009)

Moreover, the multinomial logistic analysis revealed and validated the influence of the inpatient socio-demographic characteristics on their HCSB. Patients' location, gender, age, occupation, monthly income, health insurance type, and chronic disease condition were demonstrated to be associated with the inpatient HCSB.

Compared with the male and elder patients, the female and younger patients were more likely to choose the CMCCHs for inpatient services. The possible reason was that in the rural areas, the CMCCHs were the primary institutions providing health care for children and women of child bearing age. And previous researches also showed that compared with male, female were more likely to choose higher-level HCFs. (Han, 2012; Liu & Yang, 2011)

However, the farmers, workers, and NRCMS enrollees were more likely to choose the THs rather than the county-level HCFs. This was consistent with what was mentioned above that the more convenient location and higher reimbursement rate made the THs more preferable for these groups of inpatients.

And also those suffering from chronic diseases preferred the THs rather than the county-level HCFs. The result was in accordance with the previous study in Shandong that the rural residents with chronic diseases were more likely to choose lower-level HCFs due to the higher reimbursement rate. (Jing et al., 2010)

However, in contrast to the inpatients with a monthly income above 4,000 *yuan*, the inpatients with a lower income were more likely to choose the CGMs. The result was contradicted to previous studies that patients with a higher income level were more likely to select higher level HCFs. (Jia, 2010; Li, Wang, Liu & Sun, 2016; Wang et al, 2014; Yu et al., 2006) This might be because the proportion of the patients with a monthly income above 4,000 *yuan* was too small compared with that of the patients with a lower income. Therefore, further study should try to include more patients with relatively high incomes to double check this result.

Thus, in this study, the inpatient HCSB was verified to fit in the Andersen Behavioral Model, as it was influenced by the predisposition, the ability and the need to use health care services. The predisposing factors included patient age, gender, and occupation. The enabling characteristics contained patient monthly income, health insurance type, and location of the HCFs. The need characteristic was patient chronic disease status.

According to the findings, the inpatients in rural western China chose the THs for the convenience, while those visited the county-level HCFs for the better service quality, attitude, and professional skill, equipment. Therefore, to realize universal and equitable health care, the township hospitals should improve service quality and professional skills, and the county-level HCFs should enhance their service efficiency and convenience. At the same time, efforts should be made to intensify the construction of the overall health care system in rural western China, ensure rural resident insurance coverage, advocate health education, strengthen disease cognition, and finally to improve the rational allocation of health care resources, and establish a hierarchical health care system.

Chapter 5　Result II：Inpatient satisfaction

5.1　Inpatient satisfaction with single aspect of health care services

　　Question and response distributions about the single aspect of the inpatient satisfaction are listed in Table 5-1. For all the responding inpatients, the satisfaction levels were relatively high in "communication and explanation quality of medical staff" "information provided to patients and family" "service attitude of medical staff" "professional quality of medical staff" "confidence in medical staff", and "general quality of inpatient service". However, the satisfaction levels were low in "health care expense".

　　And for each single aspect, the distributions of the satisfaction levels varied significantly among different types of the HCFs. In terms of "communication and explanation quality of medical staff" "service attitude of medical staff" "professional quality of medical staff" "confidence in medical staff" and "general quality of inpatient service", the inpatients in the THs showed relatively lower satisfaction than those in the county-level HCFs. For "information provided to patients and families" "medical equipment" and "health care expense", the inpatients in the CTCMHs and the THs showed relatively lower satisfaction. And with regards to "hospital environment", the inpatients in the CMCCHs and the THs showed relatively lower satisfaction.

Table 5-1　Inpatient satisfaction with every aspect of health care services

	CGH	CTCMH	CMCCH	TH
Communication and explanation quality of medical staff (S1) ($p=0.000^{***}$)				
Very dissatisfied	0.4%	0.8%	0.6%	0.3%
Dissatisfied	0.7%	1.5%	1.6%	1.8%
Neutral	16.6%	20.5%	14.6%	26.6%
Satisfied	38.7%	43.2%	46.7%	44.6%
Very satisfied	43.6%	34.0%	36.4%	26.8%
Information provided to patients and family (S2) ($p=0.000^{***}$)				
Very dissatisfied	0.8%	2.0%	0.5%	1.0%
Dissatisfied	1.4%	2.5%	1.3%	3.1%
Neutral	19.2%	22.9%	18.1%	28.8%
Satisfied	38.6%	44.8%	49.1%	44.9%
Very satisfied	40.0%	27.6%	31.0%	22.1%
Service attitude of medical staff (S3) ($p=0.000^{***}$)				
Very dissatisfied	3.7%	2.0%	2.5%	3.9%
Dissatisfied	2.7%	3.4%	2.9%	3.8%
Neutral	17.1%	20.6%	20.5%	23.3%
Satisfied	39.4%	44.6%	41.5%	47.1%
Very satisfied	37.1%	29.3%	32.6%	22.0%
Professional quality of medical staff (S4) ($p=0.000^{***}$)				
Very dissatisfied	1.3%	0.4%	1.1%	0.6%
Dissatisfied	1.7%	3.8%	2.2%	3.3%
Neutral	25.6%	28.8%	24.6%	39.6%
Satisfied	48.8%	49.7%	53.6%	44.7%
Very satisfied	22.6%	17.3%	18.4%	11.8%
Confidence in medical staff (S5) ($p=0.000^{***}$)				
Very dissatisfied	1.3%	2.0%	2.4%	0.9%
Dissatisfied	2.1%	2.8%	3.3%	2.9%

Continued

	CGH	CTCMH	CMCCH	TH
Neutral	22.6%	22.8%	24.0%	32.2%
Satisfied	40.5%	40.3%	46.1%	43.9%
Very satisfied	33.5%	32.1%	24.2%	20.1%
Medical equipment (S6) ($p=0.000^{***}$)				
Very dissatisfied	0.8%	1.0%	1.6%	1.4%
Dissatisfied	3.7%	7.8%	3.7%	7.0%
Neutral	32.6%	41.4%	40.4%	47.6%
Satisfied	42.4%	33.9%	38.2%	32.3%
Very satisfied	20.5%	15.9%	16.2%	11.8%
Hospital environment (S7) ($p=0.000^{***}$)				
Very dissatisfied	1.3%	1.1%	2.4%	1.2%
Dissatisfied	3.8%	5.1%	4.8%	4.6%
Neutral	34.1%	38.5%	42.4%	45.8%
Satisfied	39.6%	39.1%	36.2%	35.7%
Very satisfied	21.2%	16.2%	14.1%	12.7%
Health care expense (S8) ($p=0.000^{***}$)				
Very dissatisfied	4.2%	3.6%	2.7%	3.0%
Dissatisfied	22.0%	19.9%	14.8%	15.6%
Neutral	33.3%	44.6%	44.5%	51.1%
Satisfied	32.7%	28.0%	30.2%	19.8%
Very satisfied	7.8%	3.9%	7.8%	10.5%
General quality of inpatient service (S9) ($p=0.000^{***}$)				
Very dissatisfied	1.8%	2.5%	1.6%	1.2%
Dissatisfied	3.3%	3.2%	1.7%	2.6%
Neutral	18.9%	16.8%	23.1%	30.0%
Satisfied	54.2%	59.0%	52.6%	56.5%
Very satisfied	21.8%	18.5%	21.0%	9.6%

Note: *** $p<0.001$

5.2 Reasons for the inpatient dissatisfaction

The results regarding reasons for the inpatient dissatisfaction are shown in Table 5-2. For a clearer view of the results, Figure 5-1 is also provided.

As shown, "poor equipment" "insufficient drug supply" "tedious procedure" and "long waiting time" were the 4 aspects that the inpatients felt most dissatisfied with. And compared with those in the county-level HCFs, the inpatients in the THs showed more dissatisfaction in "poor equipment" and "insufficient drug supply". However, for "tedious procedure" and "long waiting time", relatively more patients in the CGHs showed their discontents.

Table 5-2　　　**Reasons for the inpatient dissatisfaction**

	CGH	CTCMH	CMCCH	TH
Unreasonable charge	3.5%	3.9%	2.8%	3.6%
Costly medical expense	11.1%	11.7%	9.6%	6.3%
Low professional quality	7.8%	4.6%	4.4%	11.4%
Poor equipment	20.9%	19.9%	20.6%	28.5%
Insufficient drug supply	12.9%	13.8%	13.9%	28.1%
Poor service attitude	3.8%	5.5%	2.1%	4.4%
Providing unnecessary service	3.2%	3.4%	1.6%	2.7%
Tedious procedure	19.1%	13.7%	12.7%	12.9%
Long waiting time	17.0%	14.5%	14.5%	11.5%
Others	4.9%	4.1%	9.3%	6.0%

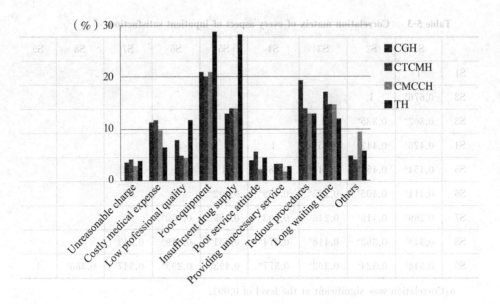

Figure 5-1　Reasons for the inpatient dissatisfaction

5.3　Overall inpatient satisfaction

5.3.1　Results of the EFA

The Cronbach's alpha was 0.854, and there was no increase in alpha when a single item was deleted. It suggested that the internal consistency of the 9 items was excellent to examine the overall inpatient satisfaction.

The inter-correlations among the items were checked and the results were presented in Table 5-3. None of the aspects correlated too highly (r＞0.9) or too lowly (r＜0.1) with the others, confirming that the EFA could be performed with the 9 items.

Table 5-3   Correlation matrix of every aspect of inpatient satisfaction

	S1	S2	S3	S4	S5	S6	S7	S8	S9
S1	1								
S2	0.676[a]	1							
S3	0.302[a]	0.335[a]	1						
S4	0.426[a]	0.442[a]	0.351[a]	1					
S5	0.454[a]	0.453[a]	0.444[a]	0.480[a]	1				
S6	0.411[a]	0.405[a]	0.225[a]	0.469[a]	0.402[a]	1			
S7	0.369[a]	0.418[a]	0.246[a]	0.503[a]	0.389[a]	0.550[a]	1		
S8	0.348[a]	0.362[a]	0.416[a]	0.374[a]	0.431[a]	0.319[a]	0.343[a]	1	
S9	0.348[a]	0.324[a]	0.392[a]	0.377[a]	0.493[a]	0.293[a]	0.347[a]	0.385[a]	1

a: Correlation was significant at the level of 0.001.

As shown in Table 5-4, the KMO measure of sampling adequacy was 0.878, and the result of Bartlett's test was 12694.653 ($p=0.000$), indicating that the sample was factorable.

Table 5-4   Results of the KMO and the Bartlett's test

Kaiser-Meyer-Olkin Measure of Sampling Adequacy		0.878
	Approx. Chi-Square	12694.653
Bartlett's Test of Sphericity	Df	36
	p	0.000

And Table 5-5 shows that all extraction communalities were greater than 0.5, indicating that the items within each domain had a very high association among them.

Table 5-5   Extraction communalities of every aspect
of inpatient satisfaction

	Initial	Extraction
S1	1.000	0.840
S2	1.000	0.826
S3	1.000	0.701

Continued

	Initial	Extraction
S4	1.000	0.589
S5	1.000	0.648
S6	1.000	0.718
S7	1.000	0.739
S8	1.000	0.773
S9	1.000	0.853

With varimax rotation and the principle of explaining as much variance as possible, three non-trivial factors representing different satisfaction subdomains were finally extracted. They totally explained 67.235% of the variance of the 9 items, and the results are shown in Table 5-6.

Table 5-6　　Eigenvalues and percentage of variance explained by EFA
for the overall inpatient satisfaction

	Initial Eigenvalues			Rotation Sums of Squared Loadings		
	Total	% of Variance	Cumulative %	Total	% of Variance	Cumulative %
S1	4.197	46.636	46.636	2.257	25.075	25.075
S2	1.019	11.323	57.958	2.039	22.656	47.731
S3	0.835	9.277	67.235	1.755	19.504	67.235
S4	0.636	7.064	74.299			
S5	0.581	6.459	80.759			
S6	0.505	5.611	86.370			
S7	0.488	5.421	91.791			
S8	0.425	4.726	96.517			
S9	0.313	3.483	100.000			

Item participations into each factor were shown in Table 5-7. Four items, including "service attitude of medical staffs" "health care expense" "confidence in medical staff" and "general quality of inpatient service", loaded onto the first factor, which reported the satisfaction with the doctor-patient relationship, health care expense, and general impression of the inpatient care. The first factor accounted for the most variance at 25.075%. Three items, "profession quality of medical staff" "medical equipment", and "hospital environment", loaded onto the second factor, which reported the satisfaction with the quality of health care, and explained 22.433% of the variance. Two items, "communication and explanation quality of medical staff" and "information provided to patients", loaded onto the third factor, which reported the satisfaction with the interpersonal skills of medical staffs and explained 19.477% of the variance.

Table 5-7 Rotated Component Matrix^a for the overall inpatient satisfaction

	Factor		
	1	2	3
S1	0.221	0.226	0.859
S2	0.230	0.256	0.841
S3	0.792	0.012	0.166
S4	0.375	0.619	0.255
S5	0.631	0.316	0.324
S6	0.124	0.801	0.232
S7	0.196	0.823	0.151
S8	0.664	0.236	0.166
S9	0.704	0.250	0.099

a: Rotation converged in 5 iterations.

The resulted factor score coefficients are presented in Table 5-8. Therefore, the formula for the three factors and the overall satisfaction are as follows:

$$F1 = -0.132 * S1 - 0.129 * S2 + 0.504 * S3 + 0.036 * S4 + 0.273 * S5 - 0.179 * S6 - 0.112 * S7 + 0.358 * S8 + 0.400 * S9$$

$$F2 = -0.154 * S1 - 0.126 * S2 - 0.245 * S3 + 0.317 * S4 - 0.012 * S5 + 0.534 * S6 + 0.559 * S7 - 0/033 * S8 - 0.011 * S9$$

$$F3 = 0.660 * S1 + 0.631 * S2 - 0.061 * S3 - 0.066 * S4 + 0.028 * S5 - 0.079 * S6 - 0.180 * S7 - 0.100 * S8 - 0.177 * S9$$

$$F_{os} = 0.090 * S1 + 0.092 * S2 + 0.088 * S3 + 0.101 * S4 + 0.106 * S5 + 0.090 * S6 + 0.094 * S7 + 0.093 * S8 + 0.094 * S9$$

Table 5-8 Component score coefficient matrix for the overall inpatient satisfaction

	Factor		
	1	2	3
S1	−0.132	−0.154	0.660
S2	−0.129	−0.126	0.631
S3	0.504	−0.245	−0.061
S4	0.036	0.317	−0.066
S5	0.273	−0.012	0.028
S6	−0.179	0.534	−0.079
S7	−0.112	0.559	−0.180
S8	0.358	−0.033	−0.100
S9	0.400	−0.011	−0.177

Internal consistency for each factor was examined using Cronbach's alpha. The alphas were 0.756, 0.806 and 0.625 for the three factors, respectively. And no substantial increases in alpha were found for any of the factors when eliminating any items.

5.3.2 Descriptive analysis for the overall satisfaction and satisfaction sub-domains

Table 5-9 presented the results of the descriptive analysis for the overall satisfaction and satisfaction sub-domains. Significant differences in satisfaction with each factor and the overall service were found among different HCFs.

Moreover, the differences in the satisfaction with each sub-domain and the overall inpatient care service among different types of HCFs were analyzed by Post Hoc test, and the results were shown in Figure 5-2 and Table 5-10. The inpatient satisfaction with Factor 1 in the county-level HCFs was statistically higher than that in the THs; for Factor 2, the inpatient satisfaction in the CGHs was significantly higher than that in other types of HCFs, and the satisfaction in the CTCMHs was significantly higher than that in the THs; for Factor 3, patient satisfaction in the CGHs and CMCCHs was significantly higher than that in the CTCMHs and the THs, while satisfaction in the CTCMs was significantly higher than that in the THs; However, for the overall satisfaction, patients in the CGHs showed the highest satisfaction, while those in the THs showed the lowest satisfaction, and the differences between satisfaction in the CTCMHs and the CMCCHs were not statistically salient.

Table 5-9   Descriptive analysis for the overall inpatient satisfaction and satisfaction sub-domains

	CGH	CTCMH	CMCCH	TH
F1 ($p = 0.002 **$)				
Max	5.72	5.68	5.92	5.65
Min	-0.41	-0.58	-1.05	0.57
Mean	3.78	3.78	3.80	3.67
SD	0.93	0.87	0.90	0.90
F2 ($p = 0.000 **$)				
Max	6.13	5.63	5.35	5.29
Min	-0.95	-0.48	0.60	-0.19
Mean	2.99	2.85	2.82	2.77
SD	0.83	0.85	0.80	0.86
F3 ($p = 0.000 **$)				
Max	4.98	5.32	4.96	5.26
Min	-0.51	-1.04	-1.22	-0.20
Mean	3.05	2.86	3.00	2.78
SD	0.80	0.82	0.80	0.82
F_{OS} ($p = 0.000 **$)				
Max	4.25	4.25	4.25	4.25
Min	1.69	1.41	2.08	1.50
Mean	3.30	3.20	3.24	3.11
SD	0.51	0.52	0.47	0.47

** $p < 0.01$, *** $p < 0.001$

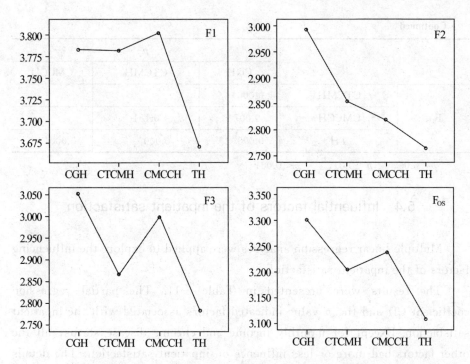

Figure 5-2　Satisfaction with each sub-domains and the
overall inpatient care services in different types of HCFs

Table 5-10　　Results of the Post Hoc test for the overall inpatient
satisfaction and satisfaction sub-domains

		p		
		CGH	CTCMH	CMCCH
	CTCMH	0.982		
F1	CMCCH	0.673	0.683	
	TH	0.002**	0.006**	0.003**
	CTCMH	0.000***		
F2	CMCCH	0.000***	0.457	
	TH	0.000***	0.019*	0.176
	CTCMH	0.000***		
F3	CMCCH	0.210	0.002**	
	TH	0.000***	0.024*	0.000***

Continued

		p		
		CGH	CTCMH	CMCCH
F_{OS}	CTCMH	0.000***		
	CMCCH	0.007**	0.181	
	TH	0.000***	0.000***	0.000***

* $p<0.05$, ** $p<0.01$, *** $p<0.001$

5.4 Influential factors of the inpatient satisfaction

Multiple linear regression analyses were applied to explore the influencing factors of the inpatient satisfaction.

The results were presented in Table 5-11. The partial regression coefficient (β) and the p value indicated factors associated with the inpatient satisfaction. Except for monthly income and chronic disease status, all the other factors had more or less influence on inpatient satisfaction. The details are as below.

For Factor 1, male inpatients ($\beta=-0.037$, $p=0.019$) showed significantly lower satisfaction. The inpatients in Guizhou ($\beta=0.087$, $p=0.000$), Inner Mongolia ($\beta=0.054$, $p=0.011$), and Shaanxi ($\beta=0.049$, $p=0.018$) showed higher satisfaction, while those in Sichuan ($\beta=-0.058$, $p=0.033$) showed lower satisfaction. Compared to the inpatients in other types of HCFs, those in the CMCCHs ($\beta=0.068$, $p=0.000$) had significantly higher satisfaction. Age was basically positively correlated with the inpatient satisfaction, with the lowest satisfaction found in the 25-34 age group ($\beta=-0.083$, $p=0.001$), secondly lowest in the 15-24 group ($\beta=-0.072$, $p=0.001$), thirdly lowest in the 35-44 group ($\beta=-0.055$, $p=0.014$), fourthly lowest in the below 14 group ($\beta=-0.053$, $p=0.003$), and fifthly lowest in the 55-64 group ($\beta=-0.040$, $p=0.043$). Occupation also had impacts on the inpatient satisfaction. Students ($\beta=0.065$, $p=0.001$) and retired people ($\beta=0.049$, $p=0.007$) had higher satisfaction. And the inpatients, who chose the corresponding HCFs for the reasons of convenient location ($\beta=-0.035$, $p=0.027$), reasonable charge ($\beta=-0.062$, $p=0.000$), professional quality of medical staffs ($\beta=-0.082$, $p=0.000$), and good service attitude ($\beta=-0.205$, $p=0.000$), were found to have lower satisfaction, while those choosing HCFs for the reason of sufficient drug supply ($\beta=0.037$, $p=0.024$) tended to have higher satisfaction.

For Factor 2, the inpatients in Inner Mongolia ($\beta=0.148$, $p=0.000$), Gansu ($\beta=0.121$, $p=0.000$), Guizhou ($\beta=0.074$, $p=0.001$), Guangxi ($\beta=0.065$, $p=0.008$), and Shaanxi ($\beta=0.045$, $p=0.033$) were shown to have higher satisfaction, and those in Tibet ($\beta=-0.049$, $p=0.008$) had lower satisfaction. Compared with the inpatients in other types of HCFs, those in the CGHs ($\beta=0.084$, $p=0.000$) had significantly higher satisfaction. And compared with the inpatients with a college diploma or above, the inpatients with less education tended to have lower satisfaction (for the illiterate, $\beta=-0.065$, $p=0.024$; for the elementary school, $\beta=-0.080$, $p=0.013$; for the middle school, $\beta=-0.064$, $p=0.029$; for the high school, $\beta=-0.070$, $p=0.002$). As for the effects of health care insurance, the inpatients enrolled in the NRCMS ($\beta=0.122$, $p=0.003$) and URRMI ($\beta=0.042$ $p=0.035$) were shown to have higher satisfaction. Moreover, the inpatients who chose the corresponding HCFs for the reasons of convenient location ($\beta=0.68$, $p=0.000$), designated HCF ($\beta=0.053$, $p=0.001$), and having an acquaintance ($\beta=0.046$, $p=0.003$) in the HCFs were found to have higher satisfaction. And those choosing the HCFs for the reasons of professional quality of medical staff ($\beta=-0.075$, $p=0.000$), advanced equipment ($\beta=-0.113$, $p=0.000$), good service attitude ($\beta=-0.034$, $p=0.040$), and having trusted doctor ($\beta=-0.043$, $p=0.005$) tended to have lower satisfaction.

For Factor 3, the inpatients in Inner Mongolia ($\beta=0.133$, $p=0.000$), Sichuan ($\beta=0.096$, $p=0.000$), Guizhou ($\beta=0.076$, $p=0.001$), Shaanxi ($\beta=0.067$, $p=0.001$), Qinghai ($\beta=0.067$, $p=0.002$), and Gansu ($\beta=0.049$, $p=0.000$) were shown to have higher satisfaction, and those in Ningxia ($\beta=-0.049$, $p=0.000$) had lower satisfaction. Compared with the other types of HCFs, the inpatients in the CGHs ($\beta=0.107$, $p=0.000$) and the CMCCHs ($\beta=0.077$, $p=0.000$) tended to have higher satisfaction. And the inpatients who chose reasonable charge ($\beta=-0.056$, $p=0.001$), professional quality of medical staffs ($\beta=-0.051$, $p=0.002$), and good service attitude ($\beta=-0.110$, $p=0.000$) as the reasons for utilizing the corresponding HCFs tended to have lower satisfaction; However, those choosing designated HCF ($\beta=0.050$, $p=0.001$), and having trusted doctor ($\beta=0.096$, $p=0.000$) were found to have higher satisfaction.

For the overall inpatient satisfaction, male inpatients ($\beta = -0.030$, $p = 0.043$) had comparatively lower satisfaction. The inpatients in Inner Mongolia ($\beta = 0.186$, $p = 0.000$), Guizhou ($\beta = 0.138$, $p = 0.000$), Shaanxi ($\beta = 0.092$, $p = 0.000$), Gansu ($\beta = 0.079$, $p = 0.001$), Xinjiang ($\beta = 0.058$, $p = 0.000$), Qinghai ($\beta = 0.042$, $p = 0.036$) had higher satisfaction, and those in Ningxia ($\beta = -0.054$, $p = 0.011$) had lower satisfaction. Compared with other types of HCFs, the inpatients in the CGHs ($\beta = 0.098$, $p = 0.000$) and the CMCCHs ($\beta = 0.097$, $p = 0.000$) tended to have higher satisfaction. Compared to the 65 and above age group, younger age groups tended to have lower satisfaction, with the lowest for the 25-34 age group ($\beta = -0.072$, $p = 0.002$), second lowest for the 15-24 group ($\beta = -0.071$, $p = 0.001$), third lowest for the 55-64 group ($\beta = -0.037$, $p = 0.043$), and fourth lowest for the below 14 group ($\beta = -0.036$, $p = 0.029$). Similar to the other satisfaction factors, the students ($\beta = 0.063$, $p = 0.001$) and retired people ($\beta = 0.046$, $p = 0.007$) also had higher overall satisfaction. And the inpatients enrolled in the NRCMS ($\beta = 0.084$, $p = 0.017$) had higher satisfaction. Moreover, the inpatients who chose reasonable charge ($\beta = -0.068$, $p = 0.000$), professional quality of medical staffs ($\beta = -0.123$, $p = 0.000$), advanced equipment ($\beta = -0.073$, $p = 0.000$), good service attitude ($\beta = -0.212$, $p = 0.00$), and having trusted doctor ($\beta = -0.084$, $p = 0.000$) as the reasons of utilizing the corresponding HCFs tended to have lower satisfaction; However, those choosing designated HCF ($\beta = 0.053$, $p = 0.000$) were found to have higher satisfaction.

Table 5-11　　Multiple linear regression results for the overall inpatient satisfaction and satisfaction sub-domains

	F1			F2		
	β	95% CI	p	β	95% CI	p
Province (reference = Yunnan)						
Inner Mongolia	0.054	0.044-0.340	0.011*	0.148	0.349-0.629	0.000***
Sichuan	-0.058	-0.266--0.011	0.033*	0.030	-0.054-0.186	0.282
Ningxia	-0.033	-0.258-0.039	0.148	-0.014	-0.183-0.097	0.550

Continued

	F1			F2		
	β	95% CI	p	β	95% CI	p
Guangxi	0.004	−0.119-0.143	0.861	0.065	0.044-0.291	0.008**
Xinjiang	0.018	−0.83-0.186	0.453	0.046	−0.002-0.250	0.055
Gansu	−0.020	−0.187-0.077	0.412	0.121	0.184-0.432	0.000***
Tibet	0.051	0.088-0.491	0.005	−0.049	−0.447-−0.066	0.008**
Guizhou	0.087	0.141-0.422	0.000***	0.074	0.091-0.356	0.001**
Shaanxi	0.049	0.031-0.327	0.018*	0.045	0.012-0.292	0.033*
Qinghai	0.004	−0.137-0.162	0.869	0.013	−0.097-0.184	0.548
Type of HCF (reference=TH)						
CGH	−0.002	−0.079-0.071	0.914	0.084	0.085-0.227	0.000***
CTCMH	0.006	−0.065-0.095	0.716	−0.001	−0.078-0.073	0.955
CMCCH	0.068	0.081-0.261	0.000***	0.024	−0.028-0.141	0.192
Gender (reference=female)						
Male	−0.037	−0.125-−0.011	0.019*	−0.002	−0.056-0.050	0.911
Age (reference≥65)						
≤14	−0.053	−0.460-−0.093	0.003**	−0.016	−0.249-0.096	0.386
15~24	−0.072	−0.334-−0.082	0.001**	−0.017	−0.165-0.073	0.445
25~34	−0.083	−0.289-−0.076	0.001**	−0.036	−0.174-0.026	0.147
35~44	−0.055	−0.236-−0.027	0.014*	0.004	−0.091-0.107	0.875
45~54	−0.030	−0.174-0.027	0.151	−0.003	−0.101-0.088	0.890
55~64	−0.040	−0.199-−0.003	0.043*	−0.008	−0.112-0.072	0.671
Education level (reference=college and above)						
Illiterate	0.041	−0.038-0.245	0.152	−0.065	−0.287-−0.020	0.024*
Elementary School	0.016	−0.095-0.159	0.618	−0.080	−0.270-−0.031	0.013*
Middle school	0.012	−0.090-0.140	0.671	−0.064	−0.228-−0.012	0.029*
High school	0.002	−0.108-0.116	0.942	−0.070	−0.269-−0.058	0.002**

Continued

	F1			F2		
	β	95% CI	p	β	95% CI	p
Occupation (reference=others)						
Farmer	0.040	−0.023-0.167	0.139	0.036	−0.028-0.150	0.181
Worker	−0.009	−0.154-0.098	0.662	−0.009	−0.145-0.092	0.656
Business/ Service	−0.032	−0.222-0.029	0.132	0.000	−0.120-0.117	0.982
Teacher/ Government staff	0.028	−0.060-0.218	0.266	0.031	−0.049-0.213	0.220
Student	0.065	0.113-0.442	0.001**	0.25	−0.053-0.257	0.199
Retired	0.049	0.071-0.451	0.007**	0.004	−0.157-0.200	0.816
Monthly income (reference=4,000 and above)						
None	−0.041	−0.231-0.071	0.298	−0.040	−0.215-0.069	0.312
1-2,000	0.010	−0.121-0.158	0.793	0.001	−0.130-0.132	0.989
2,001-4,000	0.005	−0.128-0.150	0.874	−0.028	−0.189-0.073	0.384
Health insurance (reference=no insurance)						
FMC	−0.009	−0.275-0.172	0.651	−0.001	−0.216-0.205	0.959
UEBMI	0.017	−0.125-0.217	0.597	0.058	−0.011-0.311	0.068
URBMI	0.003	−0.160-0.184	0.894	0.047	−0.011-0.311	0.072
NRCMS	0.008	−0.130-0.163	0.824	0.122	0.069-0.345	0.003**
URRMI	0.000	−0.210-0.208	0.993	0.042	0.015-0.408	0.035*
Others	0.000	−0.288-0.288	1.000	−0.010	−0.353-0.189	0.552
Chronic illness (reference=No)						
Yes	0.031	−0.001-0.125	0.052	−0.024	−0.105-0.013	0.124
Convenient location (reference=No)						
Yes	−0.035	−0.119-−0.007	0.027*	0.068	0.063-0.168	0.000***
Reasonablecharge (reference=No)						
Yes	−0.062	−0.179-−0.058	0.000***	0.002	−0.054-0.061	0.907

Continued

	F1			F2		
	β	95% CI	p	β	95% CI	p
Professional qualities (reference=No)						
Yes	−0.082	−0.231-−0.099	0.000***	−0.075	−0.204-−0.079	0.000***
Advanced equipment (reference=No)						
Yes	−0.014	−0.114-0.045	0.395	−0.113	−0.330-−0.181	0.000***
Sufficient drug supply(reference=No)						
Yes	0.037	0.017-0.239	0.024*	−0.007	−0.128-0.081	0.658
Good service attitude (reference=No)						
Yes	−0.205	−0.455-−0.332	0.000***	−0.034	−0.119-−0.003	0.040*
Designated HCF(reference=No)						
Yes	−0.002	−0.082-0.072	0.894	0.053	0.054-0.199	0.001**
Having trusted doctor (reference=No)						
Yes	−0.020	−0.132-0.026	0.189	−0.043	−0.180-−0.031	0.005**
Having acquaintance (reference=No)						
Yes	0.003	−0.107-0.126	0.870	0.046	0.058-0.278	0.003**

*p<0.05, **p<0.01, ***p<0.001.

Table 5-11   Multiple linear regression results for the overall
inpatient satisfaction and satisfaction sub-domains (continued)

	F3			F$_{os}$		
	β	95% CI	p	β	95% CI	p
Province (reference=Yunnan)						
Inner Mongolia	0.133	0.291-0.561	0.000***	0.186	0.284-0.436	0.000***
Sichuan	0.096	0.091-0.323	0.000***	0.023	−0.035-0.096	0.357
Ningxia	−0.049	−0.283-−0.013	0.032*	−0.054	−0.174-−0.022	0.011*
Guangxi	−0.026	−0.184-0.055	0.288	0.028	−0.025-0.109	0.217

Continued

	F3			F$_{OS}$		
	β	95% CI	p	β	95% CI	p
Xinjiang	0.040	−0.018-0.226	0.095	0.058	0.023-0.160	0.009**
Gansu	0.049	0.000-0.239	0.050*	0.079	0.051-0.185	0.001**
Tibet	0.012	−0.124-0.243	0.524	0.013	−0.064-0.142	0.461
Guizhou	0.076	0.093-0.349	0.001**	0.138	0.173-0.316	0.000***
Shaanxi	0.067	0.087-0.356	0.001**	0.092	0.107-0.258	0.000***
Qinghai	0.067	0.079-0.350	0.002**	0.042	0.005-0.158	0.036*
Type of HCF (reference＝TH)						
CGH	0.107	0.124-0.261	0.000***	0.098	0.068-0.145	0.000***
CTCMH	−0.015	−0.103-0.043	0.418	−0.003	−0.045-0.037	0.852
CMCCH	0.077	0.092-0.256	0.000***	0.097	0.087-0.179	0.000***
Gender (reference＝female)						
Male	−0.007	−0.063-0.039	0.647	−0.030	−0.059-−0.001	0.043*
Age (reference≥65)						
≤14	0.018	−0.081-0.252	0.316	−0.036	−0.198-−0.011	0.029*
15-24	−0.026	−0.184-0.046	0.239	−0.071	−0.178-−0.049	0.001**
25-34	0.011	−0.075-0.118	0.658	−0.072	−0.141-−0.032	0.002**
35-44	0.000	−0.095-0.096	0.990	−0.035	−0.100-0.007	0.091
45-54	0.021	−0.045-0.137	0.323	−0.012	−0.068-0.035	0.533
55-64	−0.011	−0.113-0.065	0.591	−0.037	−0.102-−0.002	0.043*
Education level (reference＝college and above)						
Illiterate	−0.034	−0.206-0.051	0.239	−0.026	−0.108-0.037	0.335
Elementary school	−0.005	−0.125-0.106	0.868	−0.038	−0.107-0.023	0.208
Middle school	−0.009	−0.121-0.088	0.758	−0.033	−0.095-0.023	0.230
High school	0.027	−0.041-0.162	0.245	−0.027	−0.093-0.021	0.216

Continued

	F3			F$_{OS}$		
	β	95% CI	p	β	95% CI	p
Occupation (reference＝others)						
Farmer	−0.050	−0.168-0.004	0.063	0.024	−0.025-0.072	0.341
Worker	−0.009	−0.139-0.090	0.674	−0.016	−0.091-0.038	0.417
Business/ Service	−0.028	−0.190-0.038	0.192	−0.036	−0.123-0.006	0.074
Teacher/ Government staff	−0.020	−0.177-0.076	0.435	0.027	−0.029-0.114	0.242
Student	0.008	−0.117-0.182	0.672	0.063	0.063-0.231	0.001**
Retired	0.020	−0.076-0.269	0.274	0.046	0.035-0.229	0.007**
Monthly income (reference＝4,000 and above)						
None	0.015	−0.111-0.163	0.713	−0.044	−0.124-0.030	0.231
1-2,000	0.018	−0.097-0.156	0.647	0.016	−0.055-0.087	0.662
2,001-4,000	0.009	−0.108-0.144	0.777	−0.008	−0.081-0.061	0.780
Health insurance (reference＝no insurance)						
FMC	0.001	−0.197-0.208	0.958	−0.006	−0.134-0.095	0.737
UEBMI	−0.002	−0.161-0.150	0.945	0.043	−0.021-0.154	0.137
URBMI	−0.004	−0.170-0.143	0.866	0.027	−0.037-0.138	0.259
NRCMS	0.029	−0.080-0.186	0.438	0.084	0.016-0.166	0.017*
URRMI	−0.014	−0.259-0.121	0.475	0.017	−0.056-0.158	0.348
Others	0.027	−0.053-0.471	0.118	0.007	−0.114-0.180	0.661
Chronic illness (reference＝No)						
Yes	−0.028	−0.109-0.005	0.074	−0.007	−0.039-0.025	0.647
Convenient location (reference＝No)						
Yes	0.026	−0.008-0.094	0.098	0.028	−0.001-0.057	0.055
Reasonable charge (reference＝No)						
Yes	−0.056	−0.152-−0.041	0.001**	−0.068	−0.102-−0.040	0.000***

Continued

	F3			F_{os}		
	β	95% CI	p	β	95% CI	p
Professional qualities (reference=No)						
Yes	−0.051	−0.153-−0.033	0.002**	−0.123	−0.170-−0.102	0.000***
Advanced equipment (reference=No)						
Yes	0.002	−0.068-0.076	0.913	−0.073	−0.138-−0.057	0.000***
Sufficient drug supply(reference=No)						
Yes	−0.006	−0.119-0.083	0.727	0.018	−0.022-0.091	0.233
Good service attitude (reference=No)						
Yes	−0.110	−0.248-−0.135	0.000***	−0.212	−0.225-−0.191	0.000***
Designated HCF(reference=No)						
Yes	0.050	0.047-0.187	0.001**	0.053	0.035-0.114	0.000***
Having trusted doctor (reference=No)						
Yes	0.096	−0.300-−0.157	0.000***	−0.084	−0.162-−0.081	0.000***
Having acquaintance (reference=No)						
Yes	0.022	−0.184-0.028	0.148	0.018	−0.022-0.097	0.218

* $p<0.05$, ** $p<0.01$, *** $p<0.001$.

5.5 Discussion

Patient satisfaction is an important and widely used indicator to evaluate health care quality and medical staff work performance. Researches on patient satisfaction evaluation could help to understand patient needs and requirements, find the shortage of health care services, so as to improve health care quality. Although many studies on patient satisfaction assessment have been carried out in China, no large-scale lucubrate study specialized in inpatient satisfaction was performed in rural western China.

In the current study, a questionnaire survey was applied to investigate the inpatient satisfaction in 11 provinces of rural western China. The questionnaire was a 5-point likert scale with 9 questions regarding different sub-aspects of patient satisfaction. For a better comparison to the other areas, five of the questions were the same as those used in the NHSS, which were satisfaction with communication and explanation quality of medical staff, information provided to patients, confidence in medical staff, hospital environment, and general quality of inpatient service.

The results shows that in terms of the 9 sub-aspects, the participating inpatients had relatively high satisfaction levels in communication and explanation quality of medical staff, information provided to patients, service attitude of medical staff, professional quality of medical staff, confidence in medical staff, and general quality of inpatient service, but low satisfaction level in health care expense. The results were basically in agreement with those of the 5th NHSS that the inpatient in rural western China had high satisfaction with the communication and explanation quality of medical staffs, information provided to patients, confidence in medical staff, general quality of inpatient service, and a medium satisfaction with the hospital environment. And same trend was also found in previous study. (Han et al., 2009; Liao et al., 2010; Shan, 2009)

Among different types of HCFs, the satisfaction aspects and levels varied significantly. The inpatients in the THs showed lower satisfaction with the communication and explanation quality of medical staff, service attitude of medical staff, professional quality of medical staff, confidence in medical staff, and general quality of inpatient service. The inpatients in the CTCMHs and the THs showed relatively lower satisfaction with the information provided to patients and families, medical equipment, and cost of care. And the inpatients in the CMCCHs and the THs showed relatively lower satisfaction with the hospital environment. These findings were partially consistent with the previous results in this study that the inpatients in rural western China chose the county-level HCFs for better service quality, attitude, and professional skill, equipment. (Duan, Niu, Xu & Zhang, 2017; Tang, Yu & Hu, 2011; Wang, Guan & Huang, 2006)

However, for the inpatient dissatisfaction, a multiple-choice question was applied to explore the dissatisfaction aspects. The results show that poor equipment, insufficient drug supply, tedious procedure, and long waiting time were the four aspects that the inpatients were most dissatisfied with. Until now, no domestic study has directly investigated this question. But according to the 5th NHSS, in rural western China, among inpatients who were dissatisfied with the general quality of inpatient service, the 4 aspects that they felt most discontented with were the costly medical expense, low professional quality, poor service attitude, and poor equipment, with dissatisfaction rates at 40.2%, 19.1%, 15.7%, and 6.1%, respectively. The reasons for the differences were that in this study, dissatisfactions of all the valid respondents were taken into account; while in the 5th NHSS, only patients discontent with the general quality of inpatient service were inquired.

And compared with those in the county-level HCFs, the inpatients in the THs showed more dissatisfaction with poor equipment and insufficient drug supply. In contrast, more inpatients in the CGHs showed their discontentment in tedious procedure and long waiting time. The finding confirmed that inpatients in this study preferred the THs due to the timely and convenient services.

The overall satisfaction with the inpatient service was investigated with the exploratory factor analysis, which extracted 3 factors representing 3 satisfaction sub-domains explaining 67.235% of the total variance. Significant differences were found in the satisfaction with each sub-domains and the overall service.

For the first sub-domain, which explained the satisfaction with doctor-patient relationship, health care expense, and general impression of the health care service, the inpatient satisfaction in the county-level HCFs was statistically higher than that in the THs.

For the second sub-domain, which explained the satisfaction with the quality of health care, the inpatient satisfaction in the CGHs were significantly higher than those in the other types of HCFs.

For the third sub-domain, which explained the satisfaction with the interpersonal sills of medical staffs, the inpatient satisfaction in the CGHs and CMCCH were significantly higher than those in the CTCMHs and THs, and satisfaction in the CTCMHs were significantly higher than those in the THs.

And, for the overall inpatient health care services, the inpatients in the CGHs showed the highest satisfaction, while those in the THs showed the lowest satisfaction, and the difference between satisfaction in the CTCMHs and the CMCCHs were not statistically obvious. The results indicate that in rural western China there were still gaps between the county-level HCFs and THs in every aspect. More efforts needed to be put into the construction of the THs in order to improve PHC coverage, provide more PHC services, promote health care quality, and further strengthen the PHC system.

Multiple linear regression analyses were applied to explore the influential factors for the inpatient satisfaction in this study. Except for monthly income and chronic disease status, all the other factors had impacts on the satisfaction factors or the overall satisfaction.

The inpatient satisfaction in different province varied significantly. The inpatients in Inner Mongolia, Guizhou, Shaanxi and Qinghai had comparatively higher satisfaction. As the GDP per capita in Inner Mongolia, Shaanxi, and Qinghai was among the top in rural western China, the results suggest that the inpatient satisfaction might be positively associated with the economic status of their residence, which was consistent with the result of previous researches. (Han et al., 2009; Qiao et al., 2010) And the results indicate that there were still evident gaps in the health resources and quality of health care services among different provinces.

Male was found to be associated with the significantly lower satisfaction with the interpersonal skill of medical staffs and the overall satisfaction. Similar results were also found in Han's study that compared with male patients, female patients had statistically significant higher satisfaction. (Han, 2012)

Age was positively correlated with the inpatient satisfaction. This was consistent with previous studies that elder patients tended to have higher satisfaction, since they might have lower expectations for the health care services, or they might not like to express their dissatisfaction. (Larsson et al., 1995; Nguyen Thi et al., 2002; Pope & Russell, 1997; Qiao et al., 2010, Rahmqvist, 2001; Wang & Jiang, 2010; Williams & Calnan, 1991; Wilde et al., 1996)

As for the patients with different occupations, students and retired people tended to have higher satisfaction. This might be because people of different occupations had different expectations for health care services.

And the patients covered by NRCMS presented higher satisfaction. The results were in accordance with former studies. (Huang, 2009; Wang &

Jiang, 2010) And to some extent, the results implies that NRCMS has made a great progress in reducing health care expense and improving health care accessibility. Therefore, the patients enrolled in NRCMS had comparatively higher satisfaction. And another reason for the higher satisfaction was because these patients might have comparatively lower expectations for health care services, for they used to have no insurance.

The reasons for choosing the corresponding HCFs also influenced the inpatient satisfactions. The inpatients choosing the corresponding HCFs for a reasonable charge, professional quality, advanced equipment, good service attitude, and having trusted doctors in the corresponding HCFs tended to have lower satisfaction, while those choosing designated HCF as the reason tended to have higher satisfaction. The results further demonstrate that health care expense, professional quality and service attitude of medical staffs, medical equipment status were of significant importance for patient satisfaction.

Chapter 6　Conclusion

This chapter is the conclusion of the findings above and puts forward policy recommendations for improvement. Moreover, the limitations of this study and the perspectives for future work are also illustrated.

The study investigated the inpatient health care seeking behavior and satisfaction in rural western China, and explored the influential factors for them.

According to the findings, in rural western China, some inpatients visited the county-level HCFs for professional skill and good service attitude, while others visited the township hospitals for timely and convenient services. The inpatient health care seeking behavior was affected by province, gender, age, occupation, monthly income, health insurance, chronic disease status, and whether the HCF had a great location, reasonable charge, professional quality, advanced equipment, sufficient drug supply, good service attitude, and acquaintances.

However, the inpatient satisfaction with each sub-domain and the overall satisfaction were higher in the county-level HCFs than those in the THs, and the inpatients in the county-level general hospitals presented the highest level. The influential factors included province, gender, age, occupation, health insurance, and whether the HCF had reasonable charge, professional quality, advanced equipment, good service attitude, and trusted doctors. The inpatients in Inner Mongolia, Guizhou, Shaanxi and Qinghai, male patients, elder patients, students, retired people, and patients enrolled in NRCMS tended to have higher satisfaction. And the patients choosing the corresponding HCFs for a reasonable charge, professional quality, advanced equipment, good service attitude, and having trusted doctors in the corresponding HCFs tended to have lower satisfaction, while those choosing designated HCFs tended to have higher satisfaction.

6.1 Policy recommendations

Fully understanding patient health care seeking behavior and providing health care according patient health care need, demand and preference help to improve patient satisfaction, and ultimately bring about the improvement in economic and social benefits of health care services. Based on from the results of the current study, four targeted recommendations are proposed for the improvement in the future studies as following：

(1) Improving professional quality of PHC system

The aim of the PHC system is to provide qualified and comprehensive health care in a cost-effective and equitable manner. Although in rural western China health care accessibility has been greatly improved by strengthening the PHC system, quality of health care services provided by the PHC facility still needs to be improved in various ways, including training adequate qualified health care workers to provide PHC services, establishing necessary infrastructure such as laboratory with necessary equipment to perform essential investigations and to confirm diagnosis, and providing essential and commonly used medicines.

(2) Simplifying procedure of health care services

Health care procedure should be simplified to facilitate residents seeking health care, especially in the secondary and tertiary hospitals. Feasible measures include establishing phone-based or web-based hospital appointment system, improving hospital information system, and providing self-service payment system.

(3) Reducing patient financial burden

The social health insurance system still needs to be improved in line with local conditions, especially for the rural areas. And on the basis of serious regulation management of the commercial health system, the integration of various insurance schemes should be done, so as to realise effective utilization of health resources and improve health care affordability.

Moreover, HCFs and relevant government departments should reduce health care expense in various ways, including giving priority to the use of essential medicines, reducing nonessential or repeated inspection, and standardizing the diagnosis and treatment procedure.

Furthermore, policy maker could promulgate some policies to support the rural or economically disadvantaged patients, such as reducing or exempting their health care expenses.

(4) Providing personalized health care service

Personalized health care service should be provided to improve patient satisfaction and health care outcomes, which means that special communication and care services will be provided, according to patients' social-demographic characteristics, health care demand and preference.

Moreover, the government should make efforts to narrow the internal gap among the rural western China, so as to meet the complicated health care needs of different rural residents.

6.2　Limitations

The results of this study some limitations.

Firstly, the planned criteria for selecting sites of HCFs and recruiting patients were the same among different areas, which did not take into consideration the economic and population differences in and among different areas. For example, in 2014, the population was 81.4 million in Sichuan, while in Tibet the population was about 3.2 million (Statistical Bureau of Sichun & NBS Survey Office in Sichuan, 2015; Tibet Autonomous Region Bureau of Statistics & Tibet General Team of Investigation under the NBS, 2015). And the GDP per capita was 26,433 *yuan* in Gansu, while in Inner Mongolia it was 71,046 *yuan* (Inner Mongolia Autonomous Regional Bureau of Statistics, 2015; Gansu Development Yearbook Editorial Board, 2015). Therefore, the data collected in this study might not be perfectly representative for the whole rural western China. Secondly, all the participants in the current study were the inpatients in the selected HCFs, so the results could not be generalized for the whole population in rural western China. For some residents, they might choose self-medication instead of seeing a doctor. Thirdly, western China is populated by Chinese minority-ethnic groups, but the current study did not take the participants' ethnicity into account. As is known, many minorities have their own medicines, such as Tibetan, Mongolian, Hui, and so on. For some people of ethnic minorities, they would like to choose the ethno-medicine rather than the regular health care service targeted in the current study. Therefore, the results of this study could not represent this group very well.

6.3 Perspectives of future work

The study focused on the inpatient health care seeking behavior and satisfaction in rural western China. Inpatient in urban areas and in eastern and central regions, as well as outpatients were out of scope in the current study, and can be investigated by repeating this research. Also, there is still a room for further study to make improvements in data collection, variable selection and questionnaire design. Additionally, the study can be repeated for the same population in the following years with the results of the present study as baseline assessment, so as to find out the progress of health care reforms. Furthermore, it will be interesting to do some comparisons among different HCFs or different areas.

References

Ajzen, I. (1985). From intentions to actions: a theory of planned behavior. In Kuhl, J. & Beckman, J. (eds.), *Action Control: From Cognition to Behavior* (pp. 11-39). Heidelberg: Springer.

Ajzen, I. (1989). Attitude structure and behavior. In Pratkanis, A. R., Beckler, S. J. & Greenwald, A. G. (eds.), *Attitude Structure and Function* (pp. 241-274). Hillsdale: Laurence Erlbaum.

Ajzen, I. (1991). The theory of planned behavior. *Organizational Behavior & Human Decision Processes*, 50(2).

Ajzen, I. & Driver, B. L. (1992). Application of the theory of planned behavior to leisure choice. *Journal of Leisure Research*, 24(3).

Ajzen, I. (2010). Perceived behavioral control, self-efficacy, locus of control, and the theory of planned behavior. *Journal of Applied Social Psychology*, 32(4).

Alabri, R. & Albalushi, A. (2014). Patient satisfaction survey as a tool towards quality improvement. *Oman Medical Journal*, 29(1).

Albarracín, D., Johnson, B. T., Fishbein, M. et al. (2001). Theories of reasoned action and planned behavior as models of condom use: a meta-analysis. *Psychological Bulletin*, 127(1).

Alden, D. L., Do, M. H. &Bhawuk, D. (2004). Client satisfaction with reproductive health-care quality: integrating business approaches to modeling and measurement. *Social Science & Medicine*, 59(11).

Aletras, V. H., Basiouri, F. N., Kontodimopoulos, N. et al. (2009). Development and psychometric assessment of a Greek-language inpatient satisfaction questionnaire. *Archives of Hellenic Medicine*, 26(1).

Andaleeb, S. S. (1998). Determinants of customer satisfaction with hospitals: a managerial model. *International Journal of Health Care Quality Assurance Incorporating Leadership In Health Services*, 11(6-7).

Andersen, R. (1968). A behavioral model of families' use of health services. *Journal of Human Resources*, 7(1).

Andersen, R. (1995). Revisiting thebehavioral model and access to medical care: does it matter? *Journal of Health & Social Behavior*, 36(1).

Andersen, R. & Newman, J. F. (2010). Societal and individual determinants of medical care utilization in the united states. *Milbank Quarterly*, 83(4).

Annandale, E. (2014). *The Sociology of Health and Medicine: A Critical Introduction*. Cambridge: Polity Press.

Anonymous,(2009). The standing conference of State Council of China adopted guidelines for furthering the Reform of Health-care System in principle. Ministry of Health of China. Retrieved December 27, 2017 from http://www. moh. gov. cn/publicfiles/business/htmlfiles/mohbgt/s3582/200901/38889.htm.

Attkisson, C. C. & Greenfield, T. K. (1999). The UCSF Client Satisfaction Scales: I. The Client Satisfaction Questionnaire-8. In M. Maruish (ed.), *The Use of Psychological Testing for Treatment Planning and Outcome Assessment*. Mahwah: Lawrence Erlbaum.

Attkisson, C. C. & Zwick, R. (1982). The client satisfaction questionnaire: psychometric properties and correlations with service utilization and psychotherapy outcome. *Evaluation & Program Planning*, 5(3).

Avis, M., Bond, M. & Arthur, A. (1997). Questioning patient satisfaction: an empirical investigation in two outpatient clinics. *Social Science & Medicine*, 44(1).

Baider, L., Everhadani, P. & Denour, A. K. (1995). The impact of culture on perceptions of patient-physician satisfaction. *Israel Journal of Medical Sciences*, 31(2-3).

Bao, Y. (2010). Analysis on factors influencing hospitalizing behavior of community residents with different insurance level in shanghai. *Chinese Journal of General Practice*, 3.

Bao, Y., Du, X. L., Zou, L. M. et al. (2010). Analysis and policy suggestion on hospitalizing intention of residents in shanghai. *Journal of Shanghai Jiaotong University*, 30(8).

Bao, Y. & Tao, M. F. (2009). Analysis on intention of visiting doctor and affecting factors in community residents of shanghai. *Chinese Journal of General Practice*, 6.

Bagozzi, R. P. (1981). Attitudes, intentions, and behavior: a test of some key hypotheses. *Journal of Personality & Social Psychology*, 41(4).

Bartlett, M. S. (1954). A note on the multiplying factors for various χ^2 approximations. *Journal of the Royal Statistical Society*, 16(2).

Bayu, B., Fasil, T. & Abrha, G. H. (2016). Health care seeking behavior in southwest ethiopia. *Plos One*, 11(9).

Bentler, P. M. & Speckart, G. (1981). Attitudes "cause" behaviors: a structural equation analysis. *Journal of Personality and Social Psychology*, 40.

Blackwell, D. L., Martinez, M. E., Gentleman, J. F. et al. (2009). Socioeconomic status and utilization of health care services in Canada and the United States: findings from a binational health survey. *Medical Care*, 47(11).

Bleich, S. N., Özaltin, E. & Murray, C. J. L. (2009). How does satisfaction with the health-care system relate to patient experience? *Bulletin of the World Health Organization*, 87(4).

Bowers, M. R., Swan, J. E. & Koehler, W. F. (1994). Whatattributes determine quality and satisfaction with health care delivery? *Health Care Manage Review*, 19(4).

Boyera, L., Cano, N., Zendjidjian, X. et al. (2009). Assessment of psychiatric inpatient satisfaction: a systematic review of self-reported instruments. *European Psychiatry*, 24(8).

Bradley, C. (1994). Handbook of psychology and diabetes: a guide to psychological measurement in diabetes research and practice. *Advances in Psychosomatic Medicine*, 17(1).

Brown, C., Barner, J., Bohman, T. et al. (2009). A multivariate test of an expanded Andersen health care utilization model for complementary and alternative medicine (CAM) use in African Americans. *Journal of Alternative and Complementary Medicine*, 15(8).

Brown, P. H. & Theoharides, C. (2010). Health-seeking behavior and hospital choice in china's new cooperative medical system. *Health Economics*, 18(S2).

Brunero, S., Lamont, S. & Fairbrother, G. (2010). Using and understanding consumer satisfaction to effect an improvement in mental health service delivery. *Journal of Psychiatric & Mental Health Nursing*, 16(3).

Carman, J. M. (1990). Consumer perceptions of service quality: an assessment of the SERVQUAL dimensions. *Journal of Retailing*, 66(1).

Carpenter, C. J. (2010). A meta-analysis of theeffectiveness of health belief model variables in predicting behavior. *Health Communication*, 25(8).

Carrhill, R. A. (2002). The measurement of patient satisfaction. *Journal of Nursing Care Quality*, 16(4).

Cattell, R. B. (1966). The scree test for the number of factors. *Multivariate Behavioral Research*, 1(2).

Center for Health Statistics and Information. (2003). *An Analysis Report of National Health Services Survey in China*, 2003. Beijing: Beijing Medical University and China Xie-he Medical University Joint Publishing House.

Center for Health Statistics and Information. (2008). *An Analysis Report of National Health Services Survey in China*, 2008. Beijing: Beijing Medical University and China Xie-he Medical University Joint Publishing House.

Center for Health Statistics and Information. (2013). *An Analysis Report of National Health Services Survey in China*, 2013. Beijing: Beijing Medical University and China Xie-he Medical University Joint Publishing House.

Charles, C., Gauld, M., Chambers, L. et al. (1994). How was your hospital stay? Patients' reports about their care in Canadian hospitals. *Canadian Medical Association Journal*, 150(11).

Chen, Y., Yao, H., Geng, ZH. et al. (2014). Research on human resources development and countermeasures in minority nationality regions of west China—Hotan, Kashgar, Kezhou data as example. *Chinese Health Service Management*, 2.

Chen, J., Du, X. P. & Xi, X. M. (2009). Analysis on satisfaction of residents to community health service held by different level medical institutions. *Chinese General Practice*, 15.

Cheng, T. M. (2008). China's latest health reforms: a conversation with Chinese health ministerChen Zhu. *Health Affairs*, 27(4).

Chinn, P. L. & Kramer, M. K. (2010). *Integrated theory and knowledge development in nursing*. St. Louis: Mosby.

Chomi, E. N., Mujinja, P. G., Enemark, U. et al. (2014). Health care seeking behaviour and utilisation in a multiple health insurance system: does insurance affiliation matter? *International Journal for Equity in Health*, 13(1).

Chowdhury, R. I., Islam, M. A., Gulshan, J. et al. (2010). Delivery complications and healthcare-seeking behaviour: the Bangladesh demographic health survey, 1999-2000. *Health & Social Care in the Community*, 15(3).

Clarkson, P., Mccrone, P., Sutherby, K. et al. (2010). Outcomes and costs of a community support worker service for the severely mentally ill. *Acta Psychiatrica Scandinavica*, 99(3).

Cleary, P. D., Fahs, M. C., Mcmullen, W. et al. (1992). Using patient reports to assess hospital treatment of persons with aids: a pilot study. *Aids Care*, 4(3).

Cleary, P. D. & Mcneil, B. J. (1988). Patient satisfaction as an indicator of quality care. *Inquiry*, 25(1).

Centers for Medicare and Medicaid Services. (2014). HCAHPS questionnaire 2014. Retrieved January 12, 2018 from http://www.hcahpsonline.org/.

Co, J. P. T., Ferris, T. G., Marino, B. L. et al. (2003). Are hospital characteristics associated with parental views of pediatric inpatient care quality? *Pediatrics*, 111(2).

Cohen, G., Forbes, J. & Garraway, M. (1996). Can different patient satisfaction survey methods yield consistent results? Comparison of three surveys. *British Medical Journal*, 313(7061).

Conner, M., Kirk, S. F., Cade, J. E. et al. (2003). Environmental influences: factors influencing a woman's decision to use dietary supplements. *Journal of Nutrition*, 133(6).

Covinsky, K. E., Rosenthal, G. E., Chren, M. M. et al. (2010). The relation between health status changes and patient satisfaction in older hospitalized medical patients. *Journal of General Internal Medicine*, 13(4).

Cronbach, L. J. (1951). Coefficient alpha and the internal structure of tests. *Psychometrika*, 16(3).

Crow, R., Gage, H., Hampson, S. et al. (2001). The measurement of satisfaction with healthcare: implications for practice from a systematic review of the literature. *Health Technology Assessment*, 6(32).

Dawson, R., Spross, J. A., Jablonski, E. S. et al. (2002). Probing the paradox of patients' satisfaction with inadequate pain management. *Journal of Pain & Symptom Management*, 23(3).

Donabedian, A. (1966). Evaluating quality of medical care. *Milbank Quarterly*, 83(4).

Doswell, W. M., Braxter, B. J., Cha, E. et al. (2011). Testing the theory of reasoned action in explaining sexual behavior among African American young teen girls. *Journal of Pediatric Nursing*, 26(6).

Duan, L., Niu, Y. D., Xu, Y. et al. (2017). Analysis of preference on selecting medical institutions of rural patients in Macheng, Hubei Province. *Chinese Health Resources*, 20(3).

Duan, Z., Pan, J. & Ren, Y. (2016). Investigation and countermeasures of medical behavior of urban patients in Sichuan Province. *Chinese Health Quality Management*, 1.

Edlund, M. J., Young, A. S., Kung, F. Y. et al. (2010). Does satisfaction reflect the technical quality of mental health care? *Health Services Research*, 38(2).

Edwards, C., Staniszewska, S. & Crichton, N. (2010). Investigation of the ways in which patients' reports of their satisfaction with healthcare are constructed. *Sociology of Health & Illness*, 26(2).

Eiman, J., Vilma, I. & Adolfo, R. (2012). Need, enabling, predisposing, and behavioral determinants of access to preventative care in Argentina: analysis of the national survey of risk factors. *Plos One*, 7(9).

Elliott, M. N., Kanouse, D. E., Edwards, C. A. et al. (2009). Components of care vary in importance for overall patient-reported experience by type of hospitalization. *Medical Care*, 47(8).

Elliott, M. N., Zaslavsky, A. M., Goldstein, E. et al. (2010). Effects of survey mode, patient mix, and nonresponse on CAHPS hospital survey scores. *Health Services Research*, 44.

Ellis, R. P., Mcinnes, D. K. & Stephenson, E. H. (2010). Inpatient and outpatient health care demand in Cairo, Egypt. *Health Economics*, 3(3).

Engardio, Peter (21 August 2005). China is a private-sector economy.

Bloomberg Businessweek.

Falvo, D. R. & Smith, J. K. (1983). Assessing residents' behavioral science skills: patients' views of physician-patient interaction. *Journal of Family Practice*, 17(3).

Festinger, L. (1957). *A Theory of Cognitive Dissonance*. Stanford: Stanford University Press.

Field, A. P. (2009). *Discovering Statistics Using SPSS (and Sex and Drugs and Rock "n" Roll)*. Los Angeles: SAGE.

Froehlich, G. W. & Welch, H. G. (1996). Meeting walk-in patients' expectations for testing effects on satisfaction. *Journal of General Internal Medicine*, 11(8).

Gansu Development Yearbook Editorial Board (2015). *Gansu Development Yearbook* 2014. Beijing: China Statistics Press.

Gao, Y., Zhou, H., Singh, N. S. et al. (2017). Progress and challenges in maternal health in western china: a countdown to 2015 national case study. *Lancet Global Health*, 5(5).

Giordano, L. A., Elliott, M. N., Goldstein, E. et al. (2010). Development, implementation, and public reporting of the HCAHPS survey. *Medical Care Research & Review*, 67(1).

Glanz, K., Lewis, F. M. & Rimer, B. K. (1997). *Health Behavior and Health Education: Theory, Research, and Practice*. San Francisco: Jossey-Bass.

Glanz, K. & Bishop, D. B. (2010). The role of behavioral science theory in development and implementation of public health interventions. *Annual Review of Public Health*, 31(1).

Glei, D. A., Goldman, N. & Rodríguez, G. (2003). Utilization of care during pregnancy in rural Guatemala: does obstetrical need matter? *Social Science & Medicine*, 57(12).

Greco, A., Steca, P., Pozzi, R. et al. (2015). The influence of illness severity on health satisfaction in patients with cardiovascular disease: the mediating role of illness perception and self-efficacy beliefs. *Behavioral Medicine*, 41(1).

Greenberg, G. A. & Rosenheck, R. A. (2004). Consumer satisfaction with inpatient mental health treatment in the department of veterans affairs.

Administration & Policy in Mental Health & Mental Health Services Research, 31(6).

Greenfield, T. K. &Attkisson, C. C. (1989). Steps toward a multifactorial satisfaction scale for primary care and mental health services. *Evaluation & Program Planning*, 12(3).

Gu, X. L., Yin, X. & Qian, D. F. (2017). Analyzing the behaviors of seeking medical services of patients with diabetes in one county and its influencing factors. *Chinese Health Service Management*, 34(7).

Guilford, J. P. & Fruchter, B. (1973). *Fundamental Statistics in Psychology and Education* (5th edn.). New York: McGraw-Hill.

Guo, Y. T. (2014). Residents' choice of medical services and its difference between urban and rural residents. *Medicine & Philosophy*, 8.

Habtom, G. K. & Ruys, P. (2007). The choice of a health care provider in Eritrea. *Health Policy*, 80(1).

Haj, H. I. E., Bahri, K., Rais, N. et al. (2013). Patient satisfaction: the importance of its measurement in improving the quality of care and services in a public paediatrics department. *Journal of Biology Agriculture & Healthcare*.

Hall, J. A. & Dornan, M. C. (1988). What patients like about their medical care and how often they are asked: a meta-analysis of the satisfaction literature. *Social Science & Medicine*, 27(9).

Hall, J. A., Milburn, M. A. & Epstein, A. M. (1993). A causal model of health status and satisfaction with medical care. *Medical Care*, 31(1).

Han, P. H., Liu, A. Q., Li, L. L. et al. (2009). The influential factors of the inpatients' satisfaction. *Chinese Nursing Management*, 9(10).

Han, Z. Y. (2012).Study on health seeking behavior and satisfaction of inpatients in rural hospital based on medical service distribution. Doctoral dissertation, Shandong University.

Hanson, K., Yip, W. C. & Hsiao, W. (2004). The impact of quality on the demand for outpatient services in Cyprus. *Health Economics*, 13(12).

Harrison, J. D., Young, J. M., Price, M. A.et al. (2009). What are the unmet supportive care needs of people with cancer? A systematic review. *Supportive Care in Cancer*, 17(8).

Hasin, M. A. A., Seeluangsawat, R. & Shareef, M. A. (2001). Statistical measures of customer satisfaction for health care quality assurance: a case study. *International Journal of Health Care Quality Assurance*, 14(1).

Haycox, A., Unsworth, L., Allen, K. et al. (1999). North Staffordshire community beds study: longitudinal evaluation of psychiatric in-patient units attached to community mental health centers 2: impact upon costs and resource use. *British Journal of Psychiatry the Journal of Mental Science*, 175(1).

Henderson, C., Phelan, M., Loftus, L. et al. (2010). Comparison of patient satisfaction with community-based vs. hospital psychiatric services. *Acta Psychiatrica Scandinavica*, 99(3).

Hesketh, T. & Zhu, W. X. (1997). Health in China: the healthcare market. *British Medical Journal*, 314(7094).

Huang, Y. (2011). The sick man of Asia: china's health crisis. *Foreign Affairs*, 90(6).

Huang Y. M. (2009). Research on patient satisfaction in the teitary-hospitals in Changsha. Doctoral dissertation, Central South University.

Inner Mongolia Autonomous Regional Bureau of Statistics. (2015). *Inner Mongolia Statistical Yearbook 2014*. Beijing: China Statistics Press.

Institute of Medicine (US) Committee on Quality of HealthCare in America. (2001). Crossing the quality chasm: a new health system for the 21st century. *Quality Management in Healthcare*, 10(4).

Janz, N. K. & Becker, M. H. (1984). The health belief model: a decade later. *Health Education Quarterly*, 11(1).

Jing,S.S, Yin, A. T., Meng, Q. Y. et al. (2010) Study on the rural chronic patients' medical treatment choice. *Chinese Health Economics*, 29(2).

Jowett, M.,Deolalikar, A. & Martinsson, P. (2004). Health insurance and treatment seeking behaviour: evidence from a low-income country. *Health Economics*, 13(9).

Jr, W. J. (1978). Effects of acquiescent response set on patient satisfaction ratings. *Medical Care*, 16(4).

Jr, W. J., Daviesavery, A. & Stewart, A. L. (1978). The measurement and meaning of patient satisfaction. *Health Medical Care Service Review*, 1(1).

Kaiser, H. F. (1960). The application of electronic computers to factor analysis. *Educational & Psychological Measurement*, 20(1).

Kaiser, H. F. (1974). An index of factorial simplicity. *Psychometrika*, 39(1).

Kamgnia, B. (2006). Use of health services in Cameroon. *International Journal of Applied Econometrics Quantitative Studies*, 3(2).

Knudsen, H. C., Vazquez-Barquero, J. L., Welcher, B. et al. (2000). Translation and cross-cultural adaptation of outcome measurements for schizophrenia. *British Journal of Psychiatry Supplement*, 177(39).

Kravitz, R. L. (1996). Patients' expectations for medical care: an expanded formulation based on review of the literature. *Medical Care Research & Review*, 53(1).

Lacaille, L. (2013). *Theory of Reasoned Action*. New York: Springer.

Lai, J. L. & Chen, R. J. (2010). A survey based on the reasonable distribution of patients under the new cooperativemedicare policy in Panyu district of Guangzhou. *Journal of Guangdong University of Foreign Studies*, 21(6).

Larsen, D. L., Attkisson, C. C., Hargreaves, W. A. et al. (1978). Assessment of client/patient satisfaction: development of a general scale. *Evaluation & Program Planning*, 2(3).

Lavy, V. & Quigley, J. M. (1993). Willingness to pay for the quality and intensity of medical care: low-income households in Ghana. Papers 94, World Bank-Living Standards Measurement.

Lebow, J. L. (1983). Research assessing consumer satisfaction with mental health treatment: a review of findings. *Evaluation & Program Planning*, 6(3).

Leese, M., Johnson, S., Slade, M. et al. (2018). User perspective on needs and satisfaction with mental health services. PRiSM psychosis study. 8. *British Journal of Psychiatry*, 173(9).

Li, F. & Jin, X. Z. (2007). Analysis on the inpatients satisfaction. *Chinese Health Quality Management*, 4.

Li, H.W., Wang, J., Liu, S. J.et al. (2016). Research and influential factors of healthcare seeking intention of outpatient among community health service institutions in Harbin. *Chinese Journal of Public Health Management*, 6.

Liao, H.Q.,Zeng, X.Y., Ren, Y.Q. et al. (2010). Research on outpatient satisfaction and its influential factors in a district of Shenzhen. *Chinese Journal of Health Statistics*, 27(4).

Like, R. &Zyzanski, S. J. (1987). Patient satisfaction with the clinical encounter: social psychological determinants. *Social Science & Medicine*, 24(4).

Linderpelz, S. U. (1982). Toward a theory of patient satisfaction. *Social Science & Medicine*, 16(5).

Liu, L. J. & Yang, W. X. (2011). Study on the first visiting medical institutions and influence factors for patients in Tianjin city. *Chinese Hospital Management*, 31(2).

Liu, W., Yang, X. F. & Zhang, J. M. (2011). Study on the elements influencing urban residents' choice behavior of medical institutions—a case of Shenyang. *Population & Development*, 4.

Lópezcevallos, D. F. & Chi, C. H. (2010). Assessing the context of health care utilization in ecuador: a spatial and multilevel analysis. *BMC Health Services Research*, 10(1).

Lupton, D. (1997). Consumerism, reflexivity and the medical encounter. *Social Science & Medicine*, 45(3).

Lupton, D., Donaldson, C. & Lloyd, P. (1991). Caveat emptor or blissful ignorance? Patients and the consumerist ethos. *Social Science & Medicine*, 33(5).

Ma, J.,Wen, J., Ren, B. B. et al. (2010). Two-weeks consultation rate and its influencing factors among rural residents with illness. *Chinese Journal of Public Health*, 26(5).

Mackian, S. (2001). A review of health seeking behaviour: problems and prospects. Retrieved December 28, 2017 from https://assets. publishing. service. gov. uk/media/57a08d1de5274a27b200163d/05-03 _ health _ seeking _ behaviour.pdf.

Marshall, G. N., Hays, R. D. &Mazel, R. (1996). Health status and satisfaction with health care: results from the medical outcomes study. *Journal of Consulting and Clinical Psychology*, 64.

Mehra, M., Bhatnagar, A. K., Rao, Y. N. et al. (2016). Prevalence and determinants of appropriate health seeking behaviour among known diabetics: results from a community-based survey. *Advances in Epidemiology*, 2014(2).

Merinder, L. B., Viuff, A. G., Laugesen, H. D. et al. (1999). Patient and relative education in community psychiatry: a randomized controlled trial regarding its effectiveness. *Social Psychiatry & Psychiatric Epidemiology*, 34(6).

Miglietta, E., Belessiotisrichards, C., Ruggeri, M. et al. (2018). Scales for assessing patient satisfaction with mental health care: a systematic review. *Journal of Psychiatric Research*, 100.

Mitchell, J. M. & Hadley, J. (1997). The effect of insurance coverage on breast cancer patients' treatment and hospital choices. *American Economic Review*, 87(2).

Montaño, D. E. & Kasprzyk, D. (2008). Theory of reasoned action, theory of planned behavior, and the integrated behavioral model. *Health Behavior*, 67-96.

Mulaik, S. A. (2009). *Foundations of Factor Analysis* (2nd edn.). Boca Raton: CRC Press.

Mummalaneni, V. & Gopalakrishna, P. (1995). Mediators vs. moderators of patient satisfaction. *Journal of Health Care Marketing*, 15(4).

Najnin, N., Bennett, C. M. & Luby, S. P. (2011). Inequalities in care-seeking for febrile illness of under-five children in urban Dhaka, Bangladesh. *Journal of Health Population & Nutrition*, 29(5).

National Bureauof Statistics of China. (2015). *China Statistical Yearbook 2015*. Beijing: China Statistics Press.

Nguyen, M. N.,Potvin, L. & Otis, J. (1997). Regular exercise in 30- to 60-year-old men: combining the stages-of-change model and the theory of planned behavior to identify determinants for targeting heart health interventions. *Journal of Community Health*, 22(4).

NguyenThi, P. L., Briançon, S., Empereur, F. et al. (2002). Factors determining inpatient satisfaction with care. *Social Science & Medicine*, 54(4).

Noar, S. M. & Zimmerman, R. S. (2005). Health behavior theory and cumulative knowledge regarding health behaviors: are we moving in the right direction? *Health Education Research*, 20(3).

Nonvignon, J., Aikins, M. K., Chinbuah, M. A. et al. (2010). Treatment choices for fevers in children under-five years in a rural ghanaian district. *Malaria Journal*, 9(1).

Norusis, M. J. (1993). *SPSS for Windows: Base System User's Guide*,

Release 5.0. Illinois: SPSS Incorporated.

Oberoi, S., Chaudhary, N., Patnaik, S. et al. (2016). Understanding health seeking behavior. *Journal of Family Medicine & Primary Care*, 5(2).

Olenja, J. (2003). Health seeking behaviour in context. *East African Medical Journal*, 80(2).

Oliver, R. L. (1993). Cognitive, affective, and attribute bases of the satisfaction response. *Journa of Consumer Research*, 20(3).

Oliver, R. L. (1997). Satisfaction: a behavioral perspective on the consumer. *Asia Pacific Journal of Management*, 2(2).

Owens, D. J. & Batchelor, C. (1996). Patient satisfaction and the elderly. *Social Science & Medicine*, 42(11).

Paddison, C. A., Abel, G. A., Roland, M. O. et al. (2015). Drivers of overall satisfaction with primary care: evidence from the English general practice patient survey. *Health Expectations*, 18(5).

Parasuraman, A., Zeithaml, V. A. & Berry, L. L. (1988). SERVQUAL: a multiple-item scale for measuring consumer perceptions of service quality. *Journal of Retailing*, 64(1).

Parkman, S., Davies, S., Leese, M. et al. (1997). Ethnic differences in satisfaction with mental health services among representative people with psychosis in south London: prism study 4. *British Journal of Psychiatry*, 171(3).

Pascoe, G. C. (1983). Patient satisfaction in primary health care: a literature review and analysis. *Evaluation & Program Planning*, 6(3).

Pinkhasov, R. M., Wong, J., Kashanian, J. et al. (2010). Are men shortchanged on health? perspective on health care utilization and health risk behavior in men and women in the united states. *Journal of Mens Health*, 6(3).

Poortaghi, S., Raiesifar, A., Bozorgzad, P. et al. (2015). Evolutionary concept analysis of health seeking behavior in nursing: a systematic review. *BMC Health Services Research*, 15(1).

Pope, C. R. & Russell, A. A. (1997). Measuring patient satisfaction: a post-visit surveyvs a general membership survey. *HMO Practice*, 11(2).

Porter, J. R. & Beuf, A. H. (1994). The effect of a racially consonant medical context on adjustment of African-American patients to physical disability. *Medical Anthropology*, 16(1-4).

Pourreza, A., Khabiri, K. R., Arab, M. et al. (2009). Health care-seeking behavior in Tehran, Iran and factors affecting it. *Journal of School of Public Health & Institute of Public Health Research*, 7(2).

Pozzi, R. (2015). The influence of illness severity on health satisfaction in patients with cardiovascular disease: the mediating role of illness perception and self-efficacy beliefs. *Behavioral Medicine*, 41(1).

Qiao, L., Liu, W. & Chen, Q. (2010). Utilization and satisfaction to community health service among residents of Beijing. *Chinese Journal of Public Health*, 7.

Rahmqvist, M. (2001). Patient satisfaction in relation to age, health status and other background factors: a model for comparisons of care units. *International Journal for Quality in Health Care Journal of the International Society for Quality in Health Care*, 13(5).

Rietveld, T. & Hout, R. V. (1993). Statistical techniques for the study of language and language behaviour. *The Journal of South African & American Studies*, 8(4).

Rodríguez, M. & Stoyanova, A. (2004). The effect of private insurance access on the choice of GP/specialist and public/private provider in Spain. *Health Economics*, 13(7).

Rosenstock, I. M. (1974). Historical origins of the health belief model. *Health Education Monographs*, 2(4).

Rosenstock, I. M., Strecher, V. J. & Becker, M. H. (1988). Social learning theory and the health belief model. *Health Education Quarterly*, 15(2).

Rous, J. J. & Hotchkiss, D. R. (2010). Estimation of the determinants of household health care expenditures in Nepal with controls for endogenous illness and provider choice. *Health Economics*, 12(6).

Rubin, H. R., Meterko, M. Nelson, E. C. et al. (1990). The patient judgments of hospital quality (PJHQ) questionnaire. *Medical Care*, 28(9 Suppl).

Ruggeri, M. (1994). Patients' and relatives' satisfaction with psychiatric services: thestate of the art of its measurement. *Social Psychiatry & Psychiatric Epidemiology*, 29(5).

Ruggeri, M. & Dall' Agnola, R. (1993). The development and use of the Verona expectations for care scale (VECS) and the Verona service satisfaction scale (VSSS) for measuring expectations and satisfaction with community-based psychiatric services in patients, relatives and professionals. *Psychological Medicine*, 23(2).

Ruggeri, M., Dall'Agnola, R., Bisoffi, G. et al. (1996). Factor analysis of the Verona service satisfaction scale-82 and development of reduced version. *International Journal of Methods in Psychiatric Research*, 6(1).

Ruggeri, M. & Greenfield, T. K. (1995). TheItalian version of the service satisfaction scale (SSS-30) adapted for community-based psychiatric patients: development, factor analysis and application. *Evaluation & Program Planning*, 18(2).

Ruggeri, M., Lasalvia, A., Bisoffi, G. et al. (2003). Satisfaction with mental health services among people with schizophrenia in five European sites: results from the epsilon study. *Schizophrenia Bulletin*, 29(2).

Ruggeri, M., Salvi, G., Perwanger, V. et al. (2006). Satisfaction with community and hospital-based emergency services amongst severely mentally ill service users: a comparison study in south-Verona and south-London. *Social Psychiatry & Psychiatric Epidemiology*, 41(4).

Sahn, D. E., Younger, S. D. & Genicot, G. (2010). The demand for health care services in rural tanzania. *Oxford Bulletin of Economics & Statistics*, 65(2).

Sepehri, A., Moshiri, S., Simpson, W. et al. (2008). Taking account of context: how important are household characteristics in explaining adult health-seeking behaviour? the case of Vietnam. *Health Policy & Planning*, 23(6).

Siddiqui, M. S., Sohag, A. A. & Siddiqui, M. K. (2011). Health seeking behavior of the people. *Professional Medical Journal*, 18.

Sinding, C. (2003). Disarmed complaints: unpacking satisfaction with end-of-life care. *Social Science & Medicine*, 57(8).

Singh, C. H. & Ladusingh, L. (2009). Correlates of inpatient healthcare seeking behavior in India. *Indian Journal of Public Health*, 53(1).

Sitzia, J. & Wood, N. (1997). Patient satisfaction: a review of issues and concepts. *Social Science & Medicine*, 45(12).

Shan, L. (2009). A study of the behavior, satisfaction level, and their determinants of insurance participants after the enactment of Shenzhen new medical insurance policy. Doctoral dissertation, Central South University.

Sheeran, P. & Taylor, S. (2010). Predicting intentions to use condoms: a meta-analysis and comparison of the theories of reasoned action and planned behavior1. *Journal of Applied Social Psychology*, 29(8).

Shipley, K.,Hilborn, B., Hansell, A. et al. (2010). Patient satisfaction: a valid index of quality of care in a psychiatric service. *Acta Psychiatrica Scandinavica*, 101(4).

Sniehotta, F. (2010). An experimental test of the theory of planned behavior. *Applied Psychology Health & Well-being*, 1(2).

Speight, J. (2005). Measuring diabetesoutcomes from the patient's perspective: appropriate selection and interpretation of psychological measures. *Hong Kong Journal of Psychiatry*, 18(1).

Spensley, J., Edwards, D. W. & White, E. (2010). Patient satisfaction and involuntary treatment. *American Journal of Orthopsychiatry*, 50(4).

Squires, A.,Bruyneel, L., Aiken, L. H. et al. (2012). Cross-cultural evaluation of the relevance of the HCAHPS survey in five European countries. *International Journal for Quality in Health Care Journal of the International Society for Quality in Health Care*, 24(5).

Stang, A. S., Hartling, L., Fera, C. et al. (2016). Quality indicators for the assessment and management of pain in the emergency department: a systematic review. *Pain Research & Management*, 19(6).

Statistical Bureau of Sichun & NBS Survey Office in Sichuan. (2015). *Sichuan Statistical Yearbook* 2014. Beijing: China Statistics Press.

Stevens, J. P. & Stevens, J. P. (2001). *Applied Multivariate Statistics for the Social Sciences* (4th Edition). Mahwah: Lawrence Erlbaum Associates.

Strecher, V. J. & Rosenstock, I. M. (1997). The health belief model. *Health Education Quarterly*, 11(1).

Tabachnick, B. G. & Fidell, L. S. (2006). *Using Multivariate Statistics* (5th edn.). Boston: Allyn & Bacon, Inc.

Tang, H. X., Yu, M. &Hu, R. Y. (2011). The advanced studies on factors of influencing residents' doctor visit. *Zhejiang Jounal of Preventive Medicine*, 23(9).

Terry, D. J., Gallois, C. & Mccamish, M. (eds.) (1995). *The Theory of Reasoned Action: Its Application to AIDS-preventive Behaviour*. Oxford:

Pergamon Press.

Tibet Autonomous Region Bureau of Statistics & Tibet General Team of Investigation under the NBS. (2015). *Tibet Statistical Yearbook 2014*. Beijing: China Statistics Press.

Vogus, T. J. & Mcclelland, L. E. (2016). When the customer is the patient: lessons from healthcare research on patient satisfaction and service quality ratings. *Human Resource Management Review*, 26(1).

Wagstaff, A., Lindelow, M., Wang, S. Y. et al. (2009). Reforming china's rural health system. *World Bank Publications*, 248.

Wang, D. et al. (2014). Survey on medical care behavior of the population with flu-like symptoms in Hefei City, AnhuiProvince. *Chinese Journal of Disease Control & Prevention*, 18(11).

Wang, H., Zhang, D.,Hou, Z. et al. (2018). Association between social health insurance and choice of hospitals among internal migrants in China: a national cross-sectional study. *BMJ Open*, 8(2).

Wang, Q., Zhang, D. &Hou, Z. (2016). Insurance coverage and socioeconomic differences in patient choice between private and public health care providers in China. *Social Science & Medicine*, 170.

Wang, Y. D., Guan, J. & Hang, L. I. (2006). Actuality of inhabitant's selection of medical institutions. *Chinese General Practice*, 9(13).

Wang, Y. Z. & Jiang, C. P. (2010). Analysis on influential factors of rural resident satisfaction with health care services.*Chinese Rural Economy*, 8.

Wang, Z. F.,Jia, J. Z., Jian, W. Y. et al. (2011). The rural primary health care of china: development and consideration. *Chinese Journal of Health Policy*, 10.

Ward, H., Mertens, T. E. & Thomas, C. (1997). Health seeking behaviour and the control of sexually transmitted disease. *Health Policy & Planning*, 12(1).

Wilde, B., Larsson, G., Larsson, M.et al. (1995). Quality of care from the elderly person's perspective: subjective importance and perceived reality. *Aging*, 7(2).

Williams, B. (1994). Patient satisfaction: a validconcept? *Social Science & Medicine*, 38(4).

Williams, B., Coyle, J. & Healy, D. (1998). The meaning of patient satisfaction: an explanation of high reported levels. *Social Science & Medicine*, 47(9).

Williams, B. & Wilkinson, G. (1995). Patient satisfactionin mental health care. evaluating an evaluative method. *British Journal of Psychiatry the Journal of Mental Science*, 166(5).

Williams, S. J. & Calnan, M. (1991). Key determinants of consumer satisfaction with general practice. *Family Practice*, 8(3).

Woodward, S., Berry, K. & Bucci, S. (2017). A systematic review of factors associated with service user satisfaction with psychiatric inpatient services. *Journal of Psychiatric Research*, 92.

Worthington, C. (2005) Patient satisfaction with health care: recent theoretical developments and implications for evaluation practice. *The Canadian Journal of Program Evaluation*, 20(3).

Xinhua News Agency (2013). *The Decision of the CPC Central Committee on Several Important Issues of Comprehensively Deepening Reform*. Beijing: People's Publishing House.

Yan, X. (2016). Research on influential factors of public's health care choice in the community medical institutions. *Chinese Health Service Management*, 2.

Yeddula, V. R. (2012). Healthcare quality: waiting room issues. Industrial and Management Systems Engineering—Dissertations and Student Research. Paper 29. Retrieved December 29, 2017 from http://digitalcommons.unl.edu/imsediss/29.

Young, J. T., Menken, J., Williams, J. et al. (2006). Who receives healthcare? Age and sex differentials in adult use of healthcare services in rural Bangladesh. *World Health & Population*, 8(2).

Yu, C., Zhao, X. & Peng, L. H. (2006). Analysis of major influential factors of choice of hospitals among urban residents. *Modern Preventive Medicine*, 33(12).

Zapka, J. G., Palmer, R. H., Hargraves, J. L. et al. (1995). Relationships of patient satisfaction with experience of system performance and health status. *Journal of Ambulatory Care Management*, 18(1).

Zhang, C. H. (2005). The study on Medical care conduct of rural residents-a survey of a rural community in the central part of China. Doctoral dissertation, Huazhong Agricultural University.

Zhang, L. (2013). Analysis of migrant workers' choice of health institutions and its influencing factors: based on the survey inNanjing. *Journal of University of Electronic Science & Technology of China : Social Sciences Edition* , 1.

Zhang, W. (2007).Research on inpatient satisfaction and its influential factors in some hospital. Doctoral dissertation, Central South University.

Zhao, W., Chen, L. & Liu, Y. (2009). Investigation on receiving medical treatment behavior of community residents and utilization of community health service centre. *Chinese Nursing Research* , 8.

Zhao, X. P., Lang, Y. & Ma, C. X. (2015). Self-reported morbidity and service utilization among migrant population in Beijing. *Capital Journal of Public Health* , 3.

Zhou, X. D., Li, L. &Hesketh, T. (2014). Health system reform in rural china: voices of healthworkers and service-users. *Social Science & Medicine* , 117(1982).

Zhou, Y. & Yan, H. E. (2008). Relevant analysis between the burden forms of medical fares and seeking medical behaviors. *Modern Preventive Medicine* , 8.

Zhou, Z. W., Mei, C. Z. & Zhang, Y. Y. (2011). Study on satisfactiondegree of outpatients in a top-notched hospital. *Modern Preventive Medicine* , 7.

Zhu, J. N., Wang, C., Zhu, L. et al. (2010). Analysis of Residents' satisfaction with health care services in Nanjing. *Chinese Journal of Public Health* , 26(5).

Zhu, L. (2010). Research on women's health problems in agriculture and animal husbandry areas of Qinghai, Gansu and Yunnan and Tibet. *Management World* , 10.

Appendix

Questionnaire for perception and satisfaction
with inpatient health care services

住院患者调查表

　　本次调查的目的是了解目前住院患者对医疗卫生服务的满意情况,探讨医疗护理质量与合格的卫生人力之间的关系,以便为提高农村地区卫生人力的存量和质量、制定卫生人力资源政策、完善管理制度提供必要的依据。根据《中华人民共和国统计法》的有关规定,本次调查将信守保密原则,所取得的数据将仅用于汇总分析,调查的信息将不会以任何形式向政府、其他机构及个人透露。

　　非常感谢您回答这份问卷,谢谢合作!

XXXXXX(学校名称)

　　机构地址:_____省(自治区)_____市_____县_____乡(镇)

　　机构全称(《医疗机构执业许可证》上登记的名称):

_____

　　组织机构代码:□□□□□□□□-□

　　(注:上面代码由调查负责人填写)

　　机构类别:□县医院　　□中医院　　□妇幼保健院　　□中心卫生院　　□一般卫生院

　　调查员(签名):_____　　填表日期:2014年_____月_____日

　　监督员(签名):_____　　填表日期:2014年_____月_____日

序号	问题及选项	回答
	患者一般情况	
1	性别：(1)男　　　(2)女	
2	年龄：_____岁	
3	文化程度： (1)没上过学　(2)小学　(3)初中　(4)高中/中专　(5)大专本科及以上	
4	职业： (1)务农　(2)务工　(3)个体　(4)政府机关及企事业单位　(5)学生 (6)退休　(7)其他	
5	您参加了哪种医疗保险(可多选)： (1)公费医疗　(2)城镇职工基本医疗保险　(3)城镇居民基本医疗保险 (4)新型农村合作医疗保险　(5)城乡居民基本医疗保险(特指) (6)商业保险　(7)其他_____　　(8)没参加	
6	您月平均收入为： (1)无收入来源　(2)2000元及以下　(3)2001～4000元　(4)4000元以上	
7	近半年内,您是否患有经医生诊断的慢性疾病? (1)是　(2)否	
	住院服务感知情况	
8	您本次住院选择该医疗机构的原因(可多选)： (1)距离近/方便　(2)收费合理　(3)技术水平高　(4)设备条件好 (5)药品丰富　(6)服务态度好　(7)定点单位　(8)有熟人 (9)有信赖医生　(10)其他	
9	住院期间,医护人员向您解释病情等问题的清晰程度如何? (1)很好　(2)好　(3)一般　(4)差　(5)很差	
10	住院期间,医生给您的关于治疗方案的意见如何? (1)很好　(2)好　(3)一般　(4)差　(5)很差	

续表

序号	问题及选项	回答
11	您认为医疗机构医务人员的服务态度如何？ (1)很好　(2)好　(3)一般　(4)差　(5)很差	
12	您觉得该医疗机构设备条件如何？ (1)很好　(2)好　(3)一般　(4)差　(5)很差	
13	您认为医院房间设施的舒适程度如何(如气味、光线、装饰及厕所的清洁程度等) (1)很好　(2)好　(3)一般　(4)差　(5)很差	
14	在接受服务过程中,您认为您所支付的医疗或药品费用如何？ (1)很贵　(2)贵　(3)一般　(4)较便宜　(5)很便宜	
15	在接受服务过程中,您认为医疗机构医务人员的技术水平如何？ (1)很好　(2)好　(3)一般　(4)差　(5)很差	
16	您对诊治您疾病的医生的信任程度如何？ (1)很不信任　(2)不太信任　(3)一般　(4)比较信任　(5)非常信任	
17	总体来说,您住院期间对该单位提供的服务的满意度如何？ (1)很不满意　(2)不太满意　(3)一般　(4)比较满意　(5)非常满意	
18	您对该机构哪些方面还不太满意？(可多选) (1)技术水平低　(2)设备条件差　(3)药品种类少　(4)服务态度差 (5)提供不必要服务　(6)收费不合理　(7)医疗费用高　(8)看病手续烦琐　(9)等候时间过长　(10)其他　(11)无	